HYPNOSIS FOR

ACUTE AND

PROCEDURAL

PAIN

MANAGEMENT:

FAVORITE METHODS OF MASTER CLINICIANS

EDITED BY MARK P. JENSEN, PHD

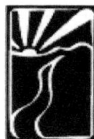

Denny Creek Press

COPYRIGHT 2019 MARK P. JENSEN

Hypnosis for Acute and Procedural Pain Management: Favorite Methods of Master Clinicians
Edition: 1st Edition
Book 3 in the *Voices of Experience*™ series.
Editor: Mark P. Jensen

ISBN# paperback: 978-1-946832-10-8
ISBN# Kindle: 978-1-946832-11-5

Library of Congress # (paperback edition only): 2018964350

Published by:
Denny Creek Press
Kirkland, Washington
Denny Creek Press, Kirkland, WA, USA
dennycreekpress@yahoo.com

Denny
Creek
Press

Cover art by Liza Brown of Modern Art Media
Interior design by Elizabeth Beeton of B10 Mediaworx

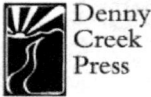

Library of Congress Cataloging-in-Publication Data

Hypnosis for Chronic Pain Management: Favorite Methods of Master Clinicians /
Mark P. Jensen, editor.
p. cm.
Includes bibliographic references
ISBN 978-1-946832-10-8 (alk. paper)
1. Hypnotism—Therapeutic Use   2. Psychotherapy

*This book is dedicated to
the clinicians who use hypnosis in
their clinical practice, with heartfelt
gratitude for your work,
bringing comfort to the world*

About the *Voices of Experience®* series

Research demonstrates that experienced hypnosis practitioners obtain better outcomes than hypnosis practitioners who are relatively new to the field. For example, Barabasz and colleagues found that the participants in a study of smoking cessation who were treated by clinicians experienced in the use of hypnosis evidenced over *four times* greater treatment response than participants who were treated by clinical psychology interns with minimal training (Barabasz et al., 1986). Although this finding may seem intuitively obvious, clinician experience has *not* been found to play a role in outcome for many other (nonhypnotic) psychological therapies (Berman & Norton, 1985; Durlak, 1979; Shapiro & Shapiro, 1982).

Thus, hypnosis outcomes appear to be particularly sensitive to the benefits of experience. This makes sense, given that hypnosis involves the creative application of specific techniques for enhancing patient readiness to accept new ideas (i.e., the hypnotic induction; Jensen, 2017), as well as the skilled use of language to develop and offer suggestions for changes in how the patient feels, thinks, or behaves. By observing the patient's immediate and longer-term response to treatment, clinicians discover and refine effective techniques and hone their use of language. Through this process they learn what works and what does not work.

Given the widespread use of hypnosis, clinicians in some regions will likely discover and develop techniques that other clinicians may not have (yet) discovered. Thus, there are master clinicians worldwide who are using effective methods that clinicians in other parts of the world may not have heard of or discovered yet.

Unfortunately, while many of the world's most experienced clinicians facilitate workshops in their own countries in which they pass on their wisdom, they do not necessarily teach at international conferences such as the tri-annual World Congress of Medical and Clinical Hypnosis (www.ishhypnosis.org). Nor is every practicing clinician able to participate in workshops that are offered around world. The purpose of the *Voices of Experience*® series is to give practicing clinicians access to the wealth of knowledge held by master clinicians throughout the world, in order to increase the ease and efficacy of treatment.

To make this information easily accessible, in the chapters contained in the series' books, the authors describe the theory or ideas that underlie their favorite hypnotic approaches and techniques. They also provide a specific transcript or scripts that illustrate the technique or approach they find useful, along with commentary. Thus, each chapter is much like having an opportunity to participate in a workshop offered by the authors. I hope and anticipate that readers will enjoy learning, and then incorporating into their practice, the wisdom and experience shared in this series.

Mark P. Jensen
Editor, *Voices of Experience*®

References

Barabasz, A. F., Baer, L., Sheehan, D. V., & Barabasz, M. (1986). A three-year follow-up of hypnosis and restricted environmental stimulation therapy for smoking.

International Journal of Clinical and Experimental Hypnosis, 34, 169-181.

Berman, J. S., & Norton, N. C. (1985). Does professional training make a therapist more effective? *Psychological Bulletin, 98,* 401-407.

Durlak, J. A. (1979). Comparative effectiveness of paraprofessional and professional helpers. *Psychological Bulletin, 86,* 80-92.

Jensen, M. P. (2017). *The art and practice of hypnotic induction: Favorite methods of master clinicians.* Kirkland, WA: Denny Creek Press.

Shapiro, D. A., & Shapiro, D. (1982). Meta-analysis of comparative therapy outcome studies: a replication and refinement. *Psychological Bulletin, 92,* 581-604.

Also available in the *Voices of Experience*® series...

Book 1. *The Art and Practice of Hypnotic Induction:
Favorite Methods of Master Clinicians*

In this volume, 11 master clinicians with over 350 years of combined clinical experience discuss the key factors necessary for effective hypnotic inductions and provide specific examples of the inductions they have found to be most effective.

Praise for *The Art and Practice of Hypnotic Induction*:

"*The Art and Practice of Hypnotic Induction* is a treasure trove of inductions with an exciting variety to accommodate patients' and clinicians' personal styles, to find the right voice." — Elvira V. Lang, MD, FSIR, FSCEH

"This is a rich read. *The Art and Practice of Hypnotic Induction* encompasses hypnotic language, the therapeutic relationship, conceptual and systemic underpinnings—the very fabric of therapy." —Leora Kuttner, PhD

"A fundamental reference for both the tyro and the expert. This entrancing collection is a must read for those interested in contemporary hypnotic practice." —Jeffrey K. Zeig, PhD

Book 2. *Hypnotic Techniques for Chronic Pain Management:*
Favorite Methods of Master Clinicians

In this volume, written by and for clinicians, 13 highly experienced physicians, psychologists, and therapists from around the world describe the hypnotic strategies they have found to be most effective for chronic pain management.

Praise for *Hypnotic Techniques for Chronic Pain Management:*

"The contributors to *Hypnotic Techniques for Chronic Pain Management* are well-known pioneers and innovative practitioners from America, Europe, and Asia. The book provides an abundance of ideas for chronic pain treatment, which even very experienced pain specialists will find inspiring and useful." — Bernhard Trenkle, Dipl Psych and President of the International Society of Hypnosis.

"*Hypnotic Techniques for Chronic Pain Management* offers an impressive number of tools for addressing the critical psychological and psychosocial issues underlying chronic pain. Examples of protocols are provided, along with descriptions of complementary and innovative clinical approaches. The pediatric perspective is also much appreciated. The reader will be left with a broad framework for treating chronic pain." — Howard Hall, PhD, Professor, University Hospitals Cleveland Medical Center.

"It is truly a pleasure and enlightening to learn from the outstanding master clinicians who contributed to *Hypnotic Techniques for Chronic Pain Management*. Each chapter provides information, ideas, and techniques that clinicians can use to help their patients (of any age) with chronic pain progress on the road to healing." — Stefan J. Friedrichsdorf, MD, Medical Director, Department of Pain Medicine, Palliative Care and Integrative Medicine, Children's Hospitals and Clinics of Minnesota

CONTRIBUTORS

Allan M. Cyna, FRCA, FANZCA, PhD
Women's and Children's Hospital
University of Adelaide
Adelaide, SA, Australia, and
Nepean Hospital, University of
Sydney
Sydney, NSW, Australia
Allan/cyna@sa.gov.au

**Roxanna Erickson-Klein, RN, LPC,
PhD**
Private Practice
Dallas, TX, USA
REricksonKlein@Gmail.com
Erickson-Klein.org

Enrico Facco, MD
University of Padua
Padua, Italy
enrico.facco@unipd.it

**Marie-Elisabeth Faymonville, MD,
PhD**
Algology-Palliative Care Department
University Hospital of Liège
Liège, Belgium
mfaymonville@chu.ulg.ac.be

Mike Gow, BDS, MFDS, RCPS
The Berkeley Clinic
Glasgow, United Kingdom
whatfearcom@hotmail.com

Mark P. Jensen, PhD, FASCH
University of Washington
Seattle, WA, USA
mjensen@uw.edu

Rob Laing, FANZCA
Women's and Children's Hospital
University of Adelaide
Adelaide, SA, Australia
rlaing@ozemail.com.au

Guy H. Montgomery, PhD
Center for Behavioral Oncology
Ichan School of Medicine at Mount
  Sinai
New York, NY, USA
guy.montgomery@mssm.edu

David R. Patterson, PhD
University of Washington
Seattle, WA, USA
davepatt@uw.edu

Audrey Vanhaudenhuyse, PhD
Algology-Palliative Care Department
University Hospital of Liège
Liège, Belgium
avanhaudenhuyse@chuliege.be

Katalin Varga, PhD
Eötvös Loránd University
Budapest, Hungary
varga.katalin@ppk.elte.hu

Lonnie K. Zeltzer, MD
Department of Pediatrics
UCLA School of Medicine
Los Angeles, CA, USA
LZeltzer@mednet.ucla.edu

CONTENTS

CHAPTER 1

Introduction

Mark P. Jensen

Acute pain is usually defined as pain that lasts less than three months (pain that persists longer than three months is chronic pain) and is attributed to a specific event or injury. It includes pain resulting from accidents (e.g., stubbed toe, muscle sprain), pain resulting from medical procedures (e.g., minor surgeries, some dental procedures), and natural processes (e.g., giving birth, muscle soreness from exercise).

Importantly, acute pain is necessary for our survival; individuals who are born without the ability experience pain do not show the usual withdrawal response to stimuli that would normally initiate pain. Because they are not able to create the experience of pain, which would warn them of the threat of physical damage, they end up experiencing repeated burns and injuries, including broken bones (Nagasako et al., 2003). As a result, these unlucky individuals have a significantly reduced life expectancy. The ability to experience pain is an important part of a healthy nervous system; pain should be viewed as a helpful friend who is looking after our safety.

However, once we are aware of an injury and are taking the necessary steps to facilitate healing, or when we are undergoing a planned medical procedure for our health that is associated with pain, acute pain loses many of its benefits. In these instances, it would be useful to be able to reduce or even eliminate the experience of pain.

Thankfully, as we evolved the ability to experience pain when nerves that detect the potential for physical damage (so-called "nociceptors") are activated, we also evolved the ability to reduce that pain experience through multiple biological mechanisms. We can reduce pain by influencing the release of chemicals in the periphery (i.e., at the site the injury); by releasing neurotransmitters in the spinal cord, where information about potential damage is initially processed; and by influencing activity in the brain, where there are multiple systems in place for decreasing (or increasing, if appropriate for our health) our experience of pain (Apkarian et al., 2005; DeLeo, 2006; Treede, 2016).

There is evidence that hypnosis and hypnotic treatments influence activity that is responsible for the creation of pain at *every level* in the nervous system, from the periphery to the central nervous system (Jensen, 2008); the mechanisms that are available to us to reduce pain are many. This is likely one of the reasons that hypnosis can be so effective for pain management.

Here, 10 master clinicians describe the hypnotic strategies and approaches they have developed and/or found to be most useful in their clinical practice for helping patients effectively manage acute pain and pain associated with medical procedures. In the first of these chapters (Chapter 2 of this book), David R. Patterson notes that there are two types of acute pain: one that is the result of an injury or acute illness, and the other that is the result of a (planned) medical procedure. Patients with acute pain that is the result of an injury may be acutely anxious, and have a difficult time concentrating. These patients are more likely to benefit from hypnotic procedures that are direct, brief, and simple. Patients who are scheduled to have a medical procedure sometime in the future can be treated before the procedure, with suggestions to link the events and cues associated with the procedure with an experience of relaxation and a sense of calm confidence. Dr. Patterson provides very clear examples of both strategies.

In Chapter 3, Katalin Varga points out that the best way to manage postoperative pain is to prevent it in the first place. She also notes that people who are about to undergo a significant medical procedure, such as a surgery, are already in a state of readiness to absorb suggestions. Because they are likely to be anxious, they may accept even neutral statements as negative suggestions. She describes how she provides these patients with a series of useful suggestions (e.g., for comfort, healing, and limited bleeding) during a pre-surgery interview. The procedure she describes involves letting the patient review and edit, as appropriate for them, the suggestions they would like to hear in a more formal hypnotic session.

Enrico Facco begins his chapter (Chapter 4) with a brief review of the history of the use of hypnosis for analgesia and a summary of the evidence supporting its efficacy for the management of surgery-related and procedural pain. He has two primary goals when using hypnosis in the management of procedural pain: a decrease in anxiety and an increase in the patient's pain threshold, although he notes that the former is easier than the latter. He provides a script for a typical hypnotic session that he would use to prepare someone for comfort during and after surgery, which includes an induction, experiencing a favorite place, suggestions for analgesia, and neglect of the operative field.

In Chapter 5, Lonnie K. Zeltzer describes a storytelling technique using imaginative involvement to help children effectively manage procedural pain and anxiety. To be most effective, clinicians need to take into account the child's developmental level (i.e., very young children need a different approach than adolescents). The goal of the storytelling strategy is to help the child become deeply involved in an experience that is inconsistent with both anxiety and pain. The themes that are most absorbing for children are often those that are exciting and involve mastery. The transcripts she offers—one for a very young child and one for an adolescent—illustrate nicely how the clinician and patient can work together to create an experience that is both enjoyable and deeply absorbing.

Hypnosis can also be used to ease labor and help make delivery safer and more comfortable for women and their newborns. In Chapter 6, Allan M. Cyna introduces the Listening, Acceptance, Utilization, Reframing, and Suggestion (LAURS) model of hypnotic communication to structure interactions with parturient women. By carefully listening to and accepting the women's experience as presented, clinicians can utilize many aspects of labor that contribute to the delivering woman's comfort. These include the "rests" that occur between contractions and the cervical dilations that occur as labor continues (signaling that the woman will soon see her baby). Treatments and interventions that could potentially be viewed as uncomfortable can be framed as experiences that will contribute to better outcomes; that is, greater comfort or increased chances for an easier birth. During labor, women are very open to suggestions, so direct, positive suggestions can be particularly useful during this time. Dr. Cyna's chapter is full of valuable tips for the use of language to enhance positive outcomes during labor and delivery.

Guy H. Montgomery is an expert in the use of hypnosis for the management of pain associated with cancer and its treatment. He begins Chapter 7 with a brief review of the evidence supporting the efficacy of hypnosis for addressing cancer-related pain. He then elegantly describes the procedures he uses to debunk myths about hypnosis and to build rapport and positive (and appropriate) outcome expectancies. He also emphasizes his careful use of language (e.g., avoiding words like "healed" and "healthy" and instead using more realistic words like "well," "comfortable," and "at ease"). The script he offers emphasizes patient choice and control, relaxation, being in a special or favorite place, and suggestions for comfort and analgesia.

Rob Laing is an anesthesiologist who uses hypnosis regularly to help his patients experience comfort during medical procedures. In his chapter (Chapter 8), after describing some general principles that can enhance the efficacy of hypnotic analgesia, he presents two transcripts that model three specific techniques that he has found particularly useful with children. These are: (1) a lived-in imagination technique that can be used to achieve multiple goals (such as distraction, relaxation, ego strengthening); (2) hypno-anesthesia suggestions for numbness for a girl about to have a venipuncture; and (3) a switch wire imagery technique for a girl undergoing burn injury debridement and dressing changes.

In Chapter 9, Roxanna Erickson-Klein describes the various hypnotic strategies that her father (Milton Erickson) used for acute pain management. His strategies often began with a clear acknowledgement of the client's or patient's experience (e.g., "That hurts awful, Robert. That hurts terrible."). Once rapport is established, the client is then ready to accept suggestions—especially suggestions that are expressly consistent with their own wishes. The cases and examples she presents from Milton Erickson's own writing illustrate how he creatively used distraction (including via storytelling), dissociation, transformation (of the sensation from pain to something else), reframing (acute pain is an opportunity to practice hypnotic skills), metaphor, time distortion, and the client's own experience ("bodily learnings") and goals, all towards the desired result of greater comfort.

Marie-Elisabeth Faymonville and Audrey Vanhaudenhuyse describe the techniques of hypnosedation for surgical patients, developed and then used in the University Hospital of Liège for over 25 years (Chapter 10). They note that the technique results not only in increased comfort but also in decreases in other symptoms related to surgery, such as anxiety and nausea, while decreasing the need for anxiolytic and analgesic medications. At the technique's core is a "Safe Place" strategy, where the patient can re-create and re-experience positive experiences.

Finally, in Chapter 11, Michael Alan Gow, a dentist, describes how he uses hypnosis to help his patients manage orofacial pain and pain associated with dental procedures. In a series of scripts, he presents clear examples of the techniques he has found most useful in his practice, including: (1) a specific rapid-induction technique, (2) his version of the "Special Place" technique, (3) a suggestion for inducing calm and a sense of control and confidence, (4) his version of glove anesthesia/analgesia, and (5) a "Comfort Dial" strategy. Although he describes these strategies in the context of managing dental procedural pain, they can all be effective for managing many acute pain problems.

Common Themes

Although the authors in this book represent clinicians from many different countries and cultures, there are a number of common themes that emerge in the chapters. The consistency of these themes argues for their importance. Interestingly, the most common themes for the treatment of acute and procedural pain differed to some degree from the most common themes from master clinicians who presented their favorite strategies for managing chronic pain (see *Hypnosis for Chronic Pain Management: Favorite Methods of Master Clinicians*, Jensen, 2018).

The themes that emerged in the chapters in this book on the management of acute pain focus on addressing anxiety, encouraging self-control and empowerment, the importance of rapport, and the common use of the "Safe Place" or "Favorite Place" techniques. The themes that emerged in the chapters by expert clinicians on chronic pain management include: (1) a consensus that chronic pain is a complex phenomenon influenced to a large degree by a number of biological, social, and psychological factors; (2) the necessity that treatments be tailored; (3) the need to target multiple domains and not just pain intensity; and (4) the importance of including suggestions that emphasize patient empowerment (Jensen, 2018). This latter theme on the importance of patient empowerment is the only one that overlaps for both pain conditions, at least in terms of the themes that are specifically discussed by different master clinicians.

Address Patient Anxiety

Almost all of the authors in this book noted that anxiety was a key co-morbid experience associated with acute and procedural pain. They therefore discussed the importance of providing information that would decrease anxiety, and they often included specific suggestions in their scripts for addressing anxiety. Perhaps the words most frequently mentioned across all of the scripts were "comfort," "relaxation," and "calm"—all three of which describe experiences that are inconsistent with a state of anxiety. For example:

- "I am calm and at peace with myself. My heart is calm and regular…" (Varga, Chapter 3).

- "You feel a pleasant sensation of relaxation… and reach a state of perfect well-being and bliss." (Facco, Chapter 4).

- "Just begin to feel a spreading sense of calm… and peace… letting go of all your cares and concerns, let them drift away, like clouds in the wind… dissipating, more and more at peace… more calm… more comfortable and secure… nothing to bother… nothing to disturb…" (Montgomery, Chapter 7).

- "And as you continue down the path you may notice some butterflies, you can realize how effortlessly they fly, as if they have let go of all their worries…" (Laing, Chapter 8).

- "These changes continue and you realize that they bring to you a certain peace of mind…" (Vanhaudenhuyse & Faymonville, Chapter 10).

Support Patient Empowerment

All pain, both acute and chronic, tends to grab the patient's attention. And because the (usually helpful and adaptive) role of pain is to protect us by motivating us to stop engaging in whatever behavior is associated with the pain, it can sometimes feel to patients as if pain is in control. Unrelenting, severe pain can make people feel powerless.

It is therefore not surprising that suggestions to empower patients are commonly included in the scripts in this book, as well as in scripts used by master clinicians for chronic pain management (Jensen, 2018). Some specific examples of the types of empowering suggestions embedded in the scripts presented are as follows:

- "I can get in touch with and activate my inner capabilities." (Varga, Chapter 3).

- "… and the excitement of knowing that you landed your spaceship expertly and gently on the moon's surface… As you walk down the stairs notice how confident you feel, how in control, as you glide down the stairs feeling relaxed, comfortable, and yet excited to have landed your spaceship so expertly on the moon… take a few moments to feel what you just accomplished… expertly going to the moon and back… in control, relaxed, and knowing that you can make this special trip whenever you want…" (Zeltzer, Chapter 5).

- "I want to assure you that no matter how deeply hypnotized you become… you will remain in complete control. … You will stay in control, even when very deeply involved in the experience of hypnosis. I will make suggestions, but it will be up to you to decide

whether you want to experience those suggestions."
(Montgomery, Chapter 7).

- *"Confident* to do the things that you *want* to do… *every
  day* feeling more and more *confident…* confident in
  yourself… confident in your *abilities…* confident in your
  talents… confident that you can become *CALM…"*
  (Gow, Chapter 10).

- "And as you walk along the rainforest path, feeling
  stronger and safer, that really happy feeling, you can
  notice how good that feels, how strong you feel, a
  feeling that you can do anything, you can achieve
  anything you want to." (Laing, Chapter 8).

Build Rapport

A close connection with patients, otherwise known as
rapport or "resonance," is known to be an important factor
contributing to the efficacy of all interventions, including
hypnotic ones (Gfeller et al., 1987; Jensen et al., 2015b; Yapko,
2012). And while rapport was often mentioned as an
important factor by master clinicians with respect to effective
hypnotic inductions (Jensen, 2017), it was not specifically
mentioned by clinicians sharing their favorite hypnotic
strategies for chronic pain management (Jensen, 2018).

On the other hand, the importance of clinician-patient
rapport was often mentioned and discussed by the authors in
this book in the context of using hypnosis for acute and
procedural pain management. Moreover, several authors
discussed the strategies they use to rapidly build rapport.

One key strategy involves making treatment patient-
centered. This is demonstrated to the patient by careful
listening and by reflecting back what the clinician hears,
thereby demonstrating an understanding of the patient's

thoughts and feelings and communicating a sense of acceptance. Allan M. Cyna (Chapter 6) does this by using the structure of LAURS (Listening, Acceptance, Utilization, Reframing, and Suggestion). Guy H. Montgomery does this by taking the time needed to ensure that he and his patients agree on what hypnosis is (and is not) and that they agree on the goals of treatment. Roxanna Erickson-Klein provided examples of how her father, Milton Erickson, was able to rapidly establish rapport by immediately acknowledging the patient's experience and primary motivation *before* making any suggestions for change. Effectively using all of these approaches requires that a clinician pay close attention to their patients.

Have Patients Experience a Safe, Special, or Favorite Place

Finally, while use of a safe, special, or favorite place is a classic hypnotic technique, it is interesting that six of the ten authors explicitly included favorite place suggestions as a component of their typical scripts for acute pain management. Examples of these, which illustrate the many similarities and some subtle differences in the use of this technique, are presented below.

- "… you can move to a terrace of a beautiful resort in a tropical isle… the sea is calm, beautifully clear… turquoise… the sand is white. … Now you are in this beautiful place, a sort of earthly paradise… where you can only have pleasant sensations…" (Facco, Chapter 4).

- "…standing at the exit of the spaceship about to go down the stairs to the moon. … Take a few moments to look around you and notice all the different aspects of the surface of the moon and all that you accomplished, flying so expertly to get here…" (Zeltzer, Chapter 5).

- "You might like to imagine being somewhere peaceful and relaxing. I like to imagine lying on a quiet beach on a warm sunny day, with a beautiful blue sky and just a few billowy white clouds floating by.… It is almost like you are really there now, enjoying your special place.… Looking off into the horizon, where the deep greens and blues of the ocean meet the white clouds and the clear blue sky. You can hear the waves crashing against the shore, the seagulls calling in the distance, perhaps your favorite song playing in the background, or just silence. Comforting. Soothing. You can feel the warmth of the sun on your skin… the cool breeze…" (Montgomery, Chapter 7).

- "As your arm comes to rest you can take yourself back to that walk in the rainforest you told me about. Look around and notice the tall trees, the beautiful flowers. Take a deep breath and smell all the rainforest smells. Listen for the sounds of insects and birds. You can look up through the trees and see the rays of light shining through. And as you see all the sights, you can step right into the forest, and really be there, taking in all the sights, the sounds, the smells…" (Laing, Chapter 8).

- "This memory, this place, slowly comes back to you and you start to see elements of it. … Slowly, the details of this wonderful place… inside your memory… come back to you, and settle into your current reality. … You find yourself slowly transported back into your safe place. As you slowly approach your peaceful place, you may hear certain sounds that invite you, deeper and deeper, back into this place. Listen closely to these sounds, maybe they're the sounds of nature... or maybe even the sound of silence" (Vanhaudenhuyse & Faymonville, Chapter 10).

- "Imagine that you are walking towards a very inviting looking door. Behind this door is a special place that your imagination is already creating for you. It may be a place that you recognize having been to before, or it may be a place entirely new. Perhaps it is a mix of both. Allow this place to be exactly the place you want it to be. It will be a safe place where you feel relaxed and at ease. You will feel freedom, peace, comfort, joy, relaxed, and rested..." (Gow, Chapter 11).

What is it about the favorite place technique that makes it so appealing to clinicians treating acute pain? The obvious first answer to this question is clear; the technique is effective—it can address a number of the factors that can contribute to pain at the same time (Jensen, 2008). For example, to the extent that patients can deeply experience themselves as being in their favorite place, they can effectively dissociate from their current environment, leaving behind "that body, back in the treatment room." Second, by being in a place where he or she feels "calm, relaxed, without a care in the world," a patient can decrease or even eliminate the negative emotions often associated with acute pain, further reducing pain intensity.

In addition, I and my colleagues have previously noted that most hypnotic suggestions require the effective use of declarative memory systems (e.g., to "remember" what it feels like to feel comfortable, calm, and relaxed; Jensen et al., 2015a). Importantly, both memory and response to hypnosis are enhanced when more of an individual's cortical neurons are firing in slow wave (e.g., theta) oscillations. Thus, by inviting the patient to experience themselves in a favorite place and to experience all of the senses associated with that place (sights, sounds, smells, sensations, and tastes), the clinician is inviting the patient to utilize and enhance those very brain oscillations most conducive to responding to hypnotic suggestions. For all of these reasons, clinicians would do well to consider incorporating favorite place suggestions as a part of hypnotic treatment.

References

Apkarian, A. V., Bushnell, M. C., Treede, R. D., & Zubieta, J. K. (2005). Human brain mechanisms of pain perception and regulation in health and disease. *European Journal of Pain, 9,* 463-484.

DeLeo, J. A. (2006). Basic science of pain. *Journal of Bone and Joint Surgery American, 88 Suppl 2,* 58-62.

Gfeller, J. D., Lynn, S. J., & Pribble, W. E. (1987). Enhancing hypnotic susceptibility:Iinterpersonal and rapport factors. *Journal of Personality and Social Psychology, 52,* 586-595.

Jensen, M. P. (2008). The neurophysiology of pain perception and hypnotic analgesia: Implications for clinical practice. *American Journal of Clinical Hypnosis, 51,* 123-148.

Jensen, M. P. (2017). *The art and practice of hypnotic induction: Favorite methods of master clinicians.* Kirkland, WA: Denny Creek Press.

Jensen, M. P. (2018). *Hypnotic techniques for chronic pain management: Favorite methods of master clinicians.* Kirkland, WA: Denny Creek Press.

Jensen, M. P., Adachi, T., & Hakimian, S. (2015a). Brain oscillations, hypnosis, and hypnotizability. *American Journal of Clinical Hypnosis, 57,* 230-253.

Jensen, M. P., Adachi, T., Tome-Pires, C., Lee, J., Osman, Z. J., & Miro, J. (2015b). Mechanisms of hypnosis: Toward the development of a biopsychosocial model. *International Journal of Clinical and Experimental Hypnosis, 63,* 34-75.

Nagasako, E. M., Oaklander, A. L., & Dworkin, R. H. (2003). Congenital insensitivity to pain: An update. *Pain, 101,* 213-219.

Treede, R. D. (2016). Gain control mechanisms in the nociceptive system. *Pain, 157,* 1199-1204.

Yapko, M. D. (2012). *Trancework: An introduction to the practice of clinical hypnosis* (4th ed.). New York, NY: Routledge.

CHAPTER 2

Hypnosis for Acute Pain

David R. Patterson

David R. Patterson is a professor of psychology in the Departments of Rehabilitation Medicine, Surgery, and Psychology at the University of Washington School of Medicine, located in Seattle, Washington, USA. He is internationally recognized for his work in the areas of hypnosis for pain control, as well as the psychology of burn and trauma injuries. Dave is the author of Clinical Hypnosis for Pain Control, *published by the APA in 2010, as well as over 150 articles and book chapters. He has been funded by the National Institutes of Health for his work using hypnosis and virtual reality for pain management since 1989. He has received numerous awards for his work in hypnosis, including the ASCH Milton Erickson Award for Scientific Excellence in Writing About Clinical Applications of Hypnosis (1997), the American Board of Psychological Hypnosis Morton Prince Award (2005), the SCEH Erica Fromm Award for Teaching in Hypnosis (2015), and the APA Psychological Hypnosis Division Distinguished Science Award (2017).*

* * *

The Two Types of Acute Pain

Acute pain differs from chronic pain in that it is directly related to a tissue injury or disease process. Acute pain is often intense, short-lived, and difficult to control. Medical and pharmacological approaches to control acute pain are typically effective and are advised as a first line of treatment. General or local anesthetics, epidural blocks, high mu receptor affinity opioid analgesics, and amnestic agents such as midazolam are among some of the approaches or agents that are often used with good results.

On the other hand, procedures and/or pharmacological approaches are sometimes not effective. Moreover, they can be expensive, have many negative side effects, and can be dangerous in many instances. Hypnosis offers a benign, cost-effective adjunct or alterative for acute pain treatment.

Acute pain is almost always a response to a trauma or illness (crisis) or is a function of a medical procedure (procedural acute pain). Both types are responsive to hypnosis, but they differ widely as to how hypnosis should be applied. In the case of crisis, the patient has a sudden onset of pain at the scene of a trauma, in the emergency room, or in the hospital. In such cases, the patient is usually in intense pain, is experiencing anxiety, and may find it challenging to provide the attention necessary for typical hypnosis. The manner in which hypnosis is applied to acute pain is different from its application to virtually any other type of clinical issue.

The second type of acute pain is procedural pain. Procedural pain is that caused by an invasive medical procedure. Examples of such include surgery, dentistry, burn care, and medical procedures (e.g., catheter insertion). Labor and delivery, although not a medical procedure, *per se*, can be considered another type of procedural pain. Procedural pain has features that make it particularly amenable to hypnosis; specifically, it usually occurs during a specified, predictable time and consequently it is possible to prepare the patient for it. What follows are two models for using hypnosis for acute pain, both of which are based on the ideas and techniques presented in my 2010 book, *Clinical Hypnosis for Pain Control* (Patterson, 2010).

Hypnosis for Acute Crisis Pain

Patients in acute pain are typically in crisis and are highly anxious. The onset of trauma or critical illness creates a fight or flight mechanism. As a result, the patient will be hypervigilant, concrete, and will often present challenges in sustaining attention. The patient's attention thus will be difficult to capture and of a limited span. Accordingly, hypnosis for acute crisis pain should usually be direct, brief, and simple. Patients are typically dependent and regressed in crisis and welcome being told what to do (e.g., "Sit down in this chair").

This presents an ideal opportunity for the clinician to use quick inductions. The role of touch becomes more useful in this type of hypnosis than in the outpatient psychotherapy situation; patients typically find touch calming.

Hypnosis for Procedural Pain

Hypnosis for procedural pain essentially uses a classical conditioning paradigm in which post-hypnotic cues for suggestion for relaxation are paired with cues that would ordinarily elicit anxiety close the procedure. Prior to the induction, the clinician determines the nature of the medical procedure as well as when and where it will be completed. An induction is completed that features deep relaxation with post-hypnotic suggestions for comfort. The relationship is given based upon the logistics of the planned procedure. The specific steps are as follows:

1. Identify the threatening medical procedure (e.g., surgery).

2. Identify events close to the procedure that will occur and may elicit anxiety (e.g., walking in the doors of the surgery clinic or unit, putting on a hospital gown, insertion of an IV needle).

3. Perform a hypnotic induction that elicits the greatest amount of deep relaxation possible.

4. Pair post-hypnotic suggestions with potential cues for anxiety (e.g., "When you put on your hospital gown, that will be the signal for your mind to create a profound sense of relaxation").

5. Alert to waking state.

Barber (1977) published a masterful script for an induction called Rapid Induction Analgesia that can be useful if the clinician substitutes cues for dental care with those that are associated with whatever procedure the clinician and the patient are preparing for.

Acute Pain Induction and Suggestions Transcript

The following induction was designed for patients in the emergency room or the intensive care unit. The assumption is that patients in these settings will be frightened, concrete, and emotionally regressed. They will not have the ability to follow complex directions or to sustain their attention for the 25-30 minutes that are required for a typical hypnotic induction. This induction is based on several quick hypnotic techniques that have been used for decades; most notably, the Spiegel eye roll technique. The general nature of this induction—for the clinician to be very direct and to take control of the process—is pretty much the opposite of the approach I use for chronic pain, in which my typical hypnotic inductions are indirect and involve non-linear suggestions as well as a cooperative approach with the patient (see Patterson, 2018).

I will use this induction primarily as an approach to calming and creating analgesia in a patient in crisis. However, I will also illustrate how this approach can be used to prepare a patient for a painful procedure. As mentioned above, however, the approach that will likely be more effective for procedural pain is one in which the clinician takes a much longer period (e.g., roughly 30 minutes) to place the patient in a deep level of relaxation before the post-hypnotic suggestions are given.

Clinician: I have been asked to see you because I understand that you are in a great amount of pain. I would like to offer you a hypnotic induction that we have been using at this hospital for over 30 years. The science behind this is remarkably strong, although our patients often do not typically think of hypnosis as having a strong scientific foundation.

> *[Hypnosis continues to carry a great deal of skepticism with it in medical communities as well as the lay public. I regard much of this skepticism to be well justified, both because lay hypnotists often make unsupported claims, and because medical professionals have been known to exaggerate the efficacy of this approach and to not acknowledge failures. In the acute setting, a short explanation of the science behind hypnosis and its proven efficacy will often be sufficient to address anxiety about hypnosis.]*

Are you willing to give this a try?

[The patient typically responds with a statement along the lines of "I will try anything at this point." If they respond affirmatively and indicate that they are willing to try hypnosis, this is the extent of my introduction. Usually, there is not time or interest in much dialogue from the patient's perspective.]

OK, I want you to follow all of my instructions carefully. I will only give you instructions that are designed to make you more comfortable. I will not make you cluck like a chicken or do anything that is not directly of benefit to you.

[Humor should only be used in this instance if the clinician feels that it is welcomed by the patient.]

[At this point the clinician places one finger on the patient's forehead above their eyes.]

OK, I want you to roll your eyes up and look at my finger. Take a deep breath...

[The clinician should allow only a momentary breath so as not to make the patient uncomfortable.]

Now, keeping your eyes rolled up, close your eye lids, let your breath out and just relax...

[At this point the clinician touches the patient's forehead with the flat of his or her hand and gently pushes back the patient's head. The touch on the forehead provides a physical cue which facilitates the quick induction. This is timed with the patient's exhalation. Often, subjects report that this type of touch is both comforting and conducive to hypnosis. This technique is based on the eye roll technique described by Spiegel and Spiegel (1978).]

Now, I am going to take your arm, and I want to see if it feels light or heavy.

[The clinician takes the arm by the wrist and gently tries to pull it up in the air. If the arm is heavy then I leave it where it is and suggest that it becomes heavier.]

That arm seems like it is nice and light so I am going to pull it up and let it float in the air.

[Obviously, the clinician follows the patient and gives this suggestion only if it is light.]

Good, let's let that arm float in the air all by itself. ... Now, after a while you may notice that the arm become heavier and starts floating downward. Just let that happen and use it as a signal from your mind. The farther your arm goes down, the deeper into hypnosis you go. So, when your arm rests on your right knee that will be a signal from your mind that you are just as relaxed as is useful to you.

[If the arm does not go down or even floats upward, the clinician just follows the patient and provides suggestions accordingly.]

Good. And now that your hand and arm are resting comfortably, I want your mind to give you a signal. When you are just as relaxed as is useful to you right now, your mind will give you a signal by allowing this finger *[touch the patient's index finger]* **to raise up in the air, seemingly under its own power.**

[This is the first of two finger signals. The signals are given using language designed to evoke dissociation. Thus, we do not say, "raise your finger," we say "your finger will raise seemingly under its own power." In many cases, the patient will not give you a finger signal. Do not be concerned if you

do not get a response. Just continue with the induction. Usually the patients that do not provide a finger signal do just as well as those that do.]

Very good. I see that your finger has signaled you. Now you can allow it to go down.

[Verbally reinforce the finger raising. Suggestions for pain relief follow.]

Now, I want to talk to a special resource in your mind. It is a part of your mind that can be of great benefit to you at times like this. I want to ask this part of your mind how it will make you feel more comfortable. I don't know how it will make you more comfortable, I only know that your body knows how to make itself more comfortable. You may not know how your mind and body will do it; only that you *will* feel more comfortable, no matter how it happens. *I do know it will happen easily and effortlessly,* without you even trying. Automatic and without effort. Now, when you know at a deep level that your body knows how it will make you feel more comfortable, your mind will signal by allowing this finger to raise a second time.

[This suggestion relies on the dissociated automaticity of hypnotic suggestion. Comfort is effortless and automatic, and we do not tell the patient how it will happen.]

Suggestions to Prepare for a Medical Procedure

Clinician: I want to talk to you now about the medical procedure you have coming up.

[Specify here whatever the patient is concerned about; e.g., surgery, childbirth, etc.]

At some point in the future you will be close to having the procedure. You will know this by signs, like going to the doctor's office *[or dental chair]* and putting on the clothes for the procedure *[if labor and delivery, you might discuss contractions occurring closer together; in any case, the clinician matches cues for the procedure here]*. Now, I want to ask the resource in your mind to do a favor for you. Somehow, you will find yourself in a profound state of comfort and relaxation for that procedure. You don't know how it will happen; I don't know how it will happen. We both just know that that procedure will be surprisingly easy and comfortable because your body will know how to do it. And when you know at a deep level that you will indeed feel comfortable during and after that procedure, and how rapidly you will heal, your mind will signal your finger to raise a second time.

[The second finger is reinforced if it rises relatively quickly; if not, then we move on.]

Now, I want you to take 30 seconds of time within your own mind to have any experience you would like. Any suggestions you want to give yourself. Allowing a deep integration to occur. Starting now...

[Allow 30 seconds.]

Now, in a few moments, but not yet—not until you are ready—I am going to start counting from five to one. With each number, you will become more alert and awake. When I reach one, your eyes will be closed but ready to open. When your mind really knows that it knows how to make you more comfortable it will signal you by allowing your eyes to open. When your eyes open, you will feel comfortable, alert, safe, and awake.

[The clinician models alertness with voice intonation while counting. The patient is allowed to keep his or her eyes closed. If groggy, the patient is instructed to close his or her eyes again and not return to alertness until they are ready.]

Final Comments

This chapter outlined hypnotic approaches for the two ways in which acute pain manifests itself. For procedural pain, hypnosis is often a simple matter of preparing the patient for the event with deep relaxation and post-hypnotic cues linked to the events preceding the surgery. For acute pain and crisis, I described a rapid induction technique that is direct but which also allows the patient to control the most important parts of the induction. Hypnosis presents opportunities for pain treatment that are unique from other psychological approaches.

References

Barber, J. (1977). Rapid induction analgesia: A clinical report. *American Journal of Clinical Hypnosis, 19*, 138-145.

Patterson, D. R. (2010). *Clinical Hypnosis for Pain Control.* Washington, DC: American Psychological Association.

Patterson, D. R. (2018). A multilayered, biopsychosocial approach to chronic pain. In M. P. Jensen (Ed.), *Hypnosis for chronic pain management: Favorite methods of master clinicians* (pp. 16-29). Kirkland, WA: Denny Creek Press.

Spiegel, H., & Spiegel, D. (1978). *Trance and Treatment: Clinical Uses of Hypnosis.* Washington, DC: American Psychiatric Press, Inc.

CHAPTER 3

Suggestive Techniques for the Management of Postoperative Pain

Katalin Varga

Dr. Katalin Varga is a professor and head of the Department of Affective Psychology at Eötvös Loránd University (ELTE), in Budapest, Hungary. She is also past president of the Hungarian Association of Hypnosis and is a board member of the International Society of Hypnosis. She was awarded a Postgraduate Fellowship of the Hungarian Academy of Sciences (1986-1990) to study the subjective experiences associated with hypnosis and the role of suggestions in critical states. She was awarded her Doctor of University degree (ELTE) in 1991, and a PhD in 1997 on comparing the subjective and behavioral effects of hypnosis. She was awarded Doctor of Science (DSc, Hungarian Academy of Sciences) in 2016 for describing phenomenological synchrony. As a member of the Budapest Laboratory of Hypnosis, she is investigating hypnosis in an interactional framework, and in this multilevel approach she is focusing on the phenomenological data. For the past 25 years she has been working with patients in a hospital setting—mostly with critically ill patients—applying suggestive and hypnotic techniques. She is the founder and professor of the postgraduate training of suggestive communication in somatic medicine, co-organized by the Hungarian Association of Hypnosis and Semmelweis University

School of Medicine, Budapest. She has published numerous articles which present her research findings regarding her clinical experience in applying suggestive techniques with the critically ill.

* * *

Patients with high levels of preoperative anxiety tend to experience more pain after surgery, as well as a greater number of complications and slower recovery (Kain et al., 2006). On the other hand, Bensen (1971) reports that in one study, 72% of appropriately prepared patients did not have any (or only slight) postoperative pain. Research data from our team demonstrate that positive suggestions without formal trance (Varga, 2017) are effective for decreasing analgesic medication intake (Schlanger et al., 2013) and reducing bleeding (Szeverényi et al., 2013, 2016; for summary see Varga, 2013).

The best way to handle postoperative pain is therefore to prevent it; one way to effectively do this is by decreasing patient anxiety before, or just after, surgery. We should understand that pain is a *signal*, telling the person that "something is wrong." Given the almost inevitable trance state of the preoperative patient, he or she will demonstrate heightened responsivity (some authors even say, vulnerability) to suggestions. As Bejenke (1996) makes clear, among the most important factors that should be addressed during the perioperative period is the patient's inability to comprehend the complexities of the illness and the procedures. Thus, for many patients, the most viable option is to accept the position of helplessness and dependence; to let go of any attempt to control the situation.

We must also not forget the "Law of Pessimistic Interpretation" (Ewin, 2011). David Cheek observed that, "If a statement can be interpreted optimistically or pessimistically, a frightened person will interpret it pessimistically" (Cheek, 1981, p. 87). According to this law, even a neutral statement or environmental element can potentially be interpreted negatively. That means that a perioperative situation is full of risk for both obvious and hidden negative suggestions. Any of these can increase the possibility that sensations will be interpreted by the patient as "pain;" that is, as a signal that "something is wrong."

Thus, the goals during surgery preparation are clear (Bejenke, 1996):

- Restore or maintain the patient's *sense of competence;*

- Increase the patient's *sense of control;*

- Foster *self-mastery* and *independence;*

- Enable the patient to *retain dignity;* and

- Include the patient as an integral and *active participant in his or her care* instead of as a passive recipient.

The critical question then becomes: How to best achieve these goals so that the patient can really collaborate/cooperate with the health care professionals in a way that fits well with the medical system?

Primary Elements of my Approach

I work as a psychologist with preoperative patients. I start the preparatory session for a surgery with the question, "How are you waiting for this operation?" The question is purposefully vague, as it allows the patient to communicate his or her key concerns. The answer will be different for each patient (e.g., "In my green pajamas," "With a fear of dying," "Alone," "Full of medication," or "Full of hope," etc.). The patient's response determines the direction of the discussion that follows.

I then ask the following question: "Have you ever considered how wonderful it is that we are not like a plastic bag?" No one has ever answered "Yes" to this question. I go on, "Plastic bags have no capacity to mend themselves... if there is a rupture. ... But the human body has this wonderful capacity to heal itself." These are truisms (statements that cannot be denied), and as a result of one surprising question, the patient is paying full attention to the "crazy" psychologist, which facilitates both rapport and an openness to clinical suggestions.

At this point I go on to describe in detail our wonderful capacity for self-healing:

Just imagine the complexity of this process. Our body locates the site where repair is needed, cleans it, transports any "garbage" from this area away, and then transports the material needed to heal and rejoin the tissues in the area... and obviously this process makes noise... it is the noise of reconstruction.

This is a basic reframing of postoperative pain. Instead of an unwanted sensation or pain, we are discussing the "noise" of a positive and forward-moving process.

Based on the recommendations of Rossi and Cheek (1988), I explain that for millions of years, while humans were living in nature, all wounds were really dirty. In such circumstances, profound bleeding was an adaptive response which helped to clean the injured area. The inflammation process cleaned it further (speaking in past tense about these "old" methods). In modern medicine, however, the areas of the body where the surgeon worked (I do not mention "wounds" again) are sterile. As a result, much, much less—if any—bleeding is needed. In addition, and because of the safety of modern medicine, much less inflammation is needed now (Szeverényi et al., 2013, 2016).

I also discuss the basic teachings of evolutionary psychology. I point out that for millions of years humankind had no remedy for actual or potential pain other than the social support of the tribe members (see Szilágyi et al., 2014, 2017). That is why the social support that the patient receives is so important: support from the family members, loved ones who are actually helping him or her or who are waiting for the patient back home; and from the professionals who are providing care—the doctors, nurses, medical assistants—everyone who is working for the patient's benefit.

This idea is an excellent example of how Bejenke (1996) connected facts (many sounds, many people, many happenings) to positive suggestions (reassuring, benefit, safe); "...as you know, there are many sounds in the operating room... and you might find it very reassuring... to hear the hustle and bustle that goes on... which lets you know that everything that is happening in that room... happens only for your benefit. Everyone in that room... is working only on your behalf... to achieve the very best for you... and to make everything safe..." (Bejenke, 1996, p. 262). The patient can also be given reframing suggestions for pain control before surgery; "...and when you feel that *pressure* underneath those bandages... as you are waking up... you can be so *relieved*... because it lets you know that your operation is completed... and that *healing* has already begun... and that you are *safe*..." (Bejenke 1996, p. 263; see also Hammond, 1990, p. 90-101).

Following this, I discuss with the patient the fact that at some level, anesthetized patients continue to hear during their operation. Thus, it can be helpful and effective to provide positive suggestions to the patient even during general anesthesia. For this I suggest the procedure that is discussed later in this chapter.

Ewin (2011) quotes Émile Coué in his summary of laws of hypnotic suggestions: "All suggestion is self suggestion." This idea is presented as a good reason why the patient is the best candidate to create suggestions for himself or herself. What I can contribute are some general ideas and topics for suggestions—a kind of "one size fits all." In response, the patient can select the suggestions, and adapt them as needed, to best fit his or her needs.

A General Approach

What follows is a standardized surgical preparation script with positive suggestions that we developed for a research project. Its efficacy has been reported (Jakubovits et al., 2011). The procedure has seven steps:

1. The patient is given a "standardized" script for an induction and suggestions to review (see the specific script, below).

2. The patient is asked to edit the script based on his or her personal wishes and goals. The patient is free to change the words, delete some sentences, or add new ones. In short, the patient is asked to tailor the script to meet his or her personal needs.

3. To maximize the efficacy of the suggestions, the patient is provided information regarding the basic rules of effective suggestions (positivity, repetition, carrot-principle, etc.; for a summary see Ewin [2011], Hammond [1990], and Varga [2015]).

4. The patient is asked to choose, from among a number of different people, whose voice the patient would like to listen to (in an audio recording) before, during, and after the operation.

5. An audio recording of the text is made by the selected person, repeating the copy as many times as needed to cover the expected time length of the operation.

6. The patient is free to listen to the audio recording as many times as she or he prefers. In some cases, a more structured approach is recommended, such as listening to the recording during the preoperative week, each day before going to sleep, and right after awakening.

7. The recording is then played during the surgery through earphones. This requires the cooperation of the anesthesiologist. Because such cooperation is not always possible, it is wise to reassure the patient that by the time of the surgery the suggestions are working "from within," even if it will not be possible to play the recording during the surgery. This is not misleading because usually, by the time of the surgery, the patient knows the text by heart, having listened to it multiple times up to that point, so the suggestions are indeed internalized at this time.

The Standard Text to be Edited by the Patient

I relax. This is an important surgery. My body and soul can work together with my surgeons. I know that I am in good hands. I trust the hospital and the competence of my doctors... I feel safe and at peace with myself. I feel that I am taken care of and am well looked after. ... I give myself over to my healers. I sleep well and I rest comfortably. Easily and comfortably...

[Establishing or strengthening rapport with the health care professionals, feeling safe and relaxed.]

Meanwhile, I see comforting images of my approaching recovery.

[Positive future orientation.]

I can get in touch with and activate my inner capabilities... My inner healing capacity gets stronger and stronger...

[Referring to the wonderful capacities of the human body. Now we have "totality"—both outside help and inner capacity.]

I am calm and I am at peace with myself. ... My heart is calm, and my heartbeat is regular; it is surprising how good I feel...

During surgery and treatments my body easily adapts to the necessary medical procedures. ... My circulation and blood pressure are appropriate at all times.

At the end of the surgery, I will wake up at the right time... with pleasant memories... and relaxed. A feeling that my healing has already started floods my consciousness. As I return to my bed, these pleasant feelings become even stronger. ... My body soon finds its inner harmony.

[Positive future and a pleasant postoperative state.]

After the surgery I recover quickly... and easily. During the post-surgery days, I wake up feeling more and more joyful... full of a refreshing, rejuvenating, healing energy.

[Repetition—a positive future and a pleasant postoperative state.]

Even if I sense anything around the area of the operation, it is an indication for me to relax… to find a comfortable position…

[Reframing pain—pain as a signal; an adaptive behavior is triggered.]

Over time, and with ease, I become even more comfortable. I completely recover…

I am surrounded by caring nurses and doctors.

[Social support.]

Every time I am examined I feel calm and more and more optimistic. After surgery I can rest easily… and I sleep well. I can move more and more easily every day.

[Healthy behavior in the future.]

All of my bodily functions return to normal…

[Restoration of automatic bodily functions, including bladder and bowel function.]

and I move more and more easily…

[Future healthy behavior.]

Every swallow is a signal to my body that my bowels can work well…

[Suggestion against vomiting.]

My digestion can be healthy, harmonious, and calm. And my appetite is better and better, so I am stronger and stronger every day…

[Restoration of vegetative functions.]

And I have more and more inner energy. My body knows how to recover fully.

[Repetition—a positive future and a pleasant postoperative state.]

I cough if I need to clear my throat. My blood circulation as well as everything else adjusts exactly to what is needed for my complete recovery.

[Restoration of vegetative functions.]

The surgical site is healing as well. It will continue to heal, all on its own. It knows what to do to get perfectly well.

The scar will be a proud reminder of what I will have been through.

[Future orientation.]

I feel better and better every day; stronger and stronger; and more and more positive. I am patient and happy. I am open to every positive influence that can promote my recovery... and I can protect myself from any negativity.

[Protection from negative suggestions as recommended by Cheek, (1960)]

Near and distant acts of kindness and attentiveness give me energy.

[Social support.]

They multiply the healing power of my body and the efficacy of any treatments I am receiving.

I can find just the right body-soul balance. I can savor and enjoy the small pleasures of life; a fine piece of clothing, delicious food, a kind smile.

[Future orientation.]

I feel stronger and healthier every day. Stronger and healthier. My recovery is fast and complete. My recovery is fast and complete.

Case Illustration

A 37-year-old patient contacted me asking for help as she prepared for her third delivery. It turned out that she had had an operation at the eighth gestational week, due to a gastro-intestinal tumor. It is worth noting that she "discovered" the tumor in her imagination while practicing autogenic training (that she learned from me 10 years before). The histology analysis later proved one single (!) malignant cell.

As might be expected, she found the operation that was performed during her pregnancy to be extremely stressful. Unfortunately, due to a wound disruption, a reoperation was needed. She also reported a traumatizing interaction with the oncology doctor. Thus, overall, this series of interventions was a very bad experience for her.

Fortunately, a healthy baby was born in a normal delivery when the baby was due. When she contacted me following the delivery, she told me she wanted to discuss the stressful event and to lose weight. The otherwise bright and pleasant woman presented as being somewhat unkempt and overweight.

During therapy, it became apparent that she wanted to avoid further oncology care and that she was not ready for the reconstructive operation that was recommended. Because she had suffered a great deal both physically and psychologically during and after the previous surgical procedures, she wanted to avoid this experience again.

We discussed that both follow-up care with an oncologist and the reconstructive operation were important for her health. I recommended a new oncologist who had better communication skills. We also began the process of preparing for the reconstructive abdominal surgery (which was to fix a hernia which would allow her to remove a hernia truss she had to wear continuously); to prepare her to be ready to "welcome" a surgical mesh in her abdomen.

During the preparation we followed the procedure described above. Focusing on the successful side of the original story, we reframed the time surrounding her previous operation as a time during which, "...your body was busy protecting your baby, who was born in good health. At that time, you did not have enough attention and energy to prevent some of the negative outcomes."

This suggestion was given to her to emphasize (1) the "wisdom" of her body in allocating the available energy to the most important goal (i.e., a healthy baby) and (2) to restore faith in the doctors (i.e., to not blame them for the negative outcomes of the previous operation). I also reinforced that she has very good communication with her own body, given her ability to discover one single malignant cell in her intestine. Thus, her self-controlled trance state proved to be very effective; we could utilize this special capacity this time as well.

Following this, she was given the standardized text and invited to tailor it to her needs. Her edits to the text can be seen in the appendix to this chapter.

She chose to hear my voice on the audio recording. She then listened to the recording repeatedly for several weeks before the operation. Whenever she started to feel anxious or wanted to escape from bad memories of the previous surgery, she immersed herself in an altered state; listening to and focusing on the self-tailored suggestions.

The operation went very well. She described the postoperative period as follows:

"Looking back I do not remember any pain. The mobility also was smooth. All in all, the postoperative time was very quick, smooth, and without any problem. I could go home quickly. I could have gone even earlier, but the doctor asked, due to the antecedents, for the sake of security I should stay for the weekend. I really remember that everything was good and easy at the hospital. Nothing else." (Personal email to the author, quoted with permission.)

At our follow-up session after the reconstructive operation, she presented as an elegant, friendly, and happy woman. She presents this way still, at 7 years follow-up.

Conclusion

With this approach, the patient took an active role; she is truly self-managing her responses and taking care of herself. She made several key decisions (e.g., editing the text, choosing the voice to hear in the recording), which gave her real control over the process. She tailored the suggestions to her special needs, so everything was personalized. This directly addressed the empowering principles outlined by Bejenke (1996). This self-tailoring process is an excellent way to make the approach fit the special characters and personality traits of a variety of patients (Kessler & Dane, 1996; Kessler, 1997).

This is a process that involves both the trance state of the patient, and a high level of cognitive function, as the patient edits the suggestions and takes into consideration her personal memories and the meaning she attributes to the situation (Jensen, 2008). The texts offers various coping strategies and healthy behavioral and vegetative patterns (e.g., eating, movement; Evans & Richardson, 1990). In addition to the specific beneficial effects of the suggestions, the audio recording serves as a type of social support which can provide special "company" to address the loneliness of a medical procedure (Couture & Bennett, 1990).

The technique is not restricted to the actual surgery time, as it extends its effects to the pre- and postoperative periods. All these perioperative phases can be considered as especially vulnerable times when the patient is particularly responsive to suggestions (Barber, 1990; Bennett et al., 1988; Hammond, 1990). Some authors stress that the preparation should start six to eight weeks before the surgery and should extend through rehabilitation (Wallace, 1987).

The unfavorable and/or psychologically traumatic experiences during surgery (e.g., as occurred in the case example described here during her previous surgery) can deeply influence the postoperative state, increasing pain as well as the consumption of analgesics (Wise et al., 1978). The overall aim of hypnotic preparation is to set the patient's anxiety and tension to an optimal level (i.e., not completely zero, because some "worry work" may be needed to adapt to the stress of operation [Averill, 1973]).

The case presented also illustrates how a difficult, emotionally or physically painful medical intervention can have a negative impact on the patient's whole personality. And it shows how a well-prepared and positive surgical experience can bring positive results: a preparation which results in a procedure that empowers the patient, gives her a sense of competence and control, and allows her to retain her dignity and be an active participant in her care.

Acknowledgement

The preparation of this Chapter was supported by OTKA K 109187 grant to Éva I. Bányai. In addition, the author would like to express her appreciation to Márta Zakó for her invaluable help in the preparation of this chapter.

References

Averill, J. R. (1973). Personal control over aversive stimuli and its relationship to stress. *Psychological Bulletin, 80,* 286-303.

Barber, J. (1990). Examples of preoperative suggestions. In D. C. Hammond (Ed.), *Hypnotic suggestions and metaphors* (p. 98). New York, NY: WW Norton & Company.

Bennett, H. L., DeMorris, K. A., & Willits, N. H. (1988). Acquisition of auditory information during different periods of general anesthesia. *Anesthesia & Analgesia, 67,* S1-S266.

Bejenke, C. J. (1996). Painful medical procedures. In J. Barber (Ed), *Hypnosis and suggestion in the treatment of pain* (pp. 209-265). New York, NY: WW Norton and Company.

Bensen, V. B. (1971). One hundred cases of post-anesthetic suggestion in the recovery room *American Journal of Clinical Hypnosis, 14,* 9-15.

Cheek, D. B. (1960). Use of preoperative hypnosis to protect patients from careless conversation (during anesthesia). *American Journal of Clinical Hypnosis, 3,* 101-102.

Cheek, D. B. (1981). Awareness of meaningful sounds under general anesthesia: Considerations and a review of the literature 1959-1979. In H. J. Wain (Ed.), *Theoretical and clinical aspects of hypnosis* (p. 87-106). Miami, FL: Symposia Specialists.

Couture, L. J., Bennett, H. L. (1990). Multi-modal content analysis of post-anesthetic hypnotic regressions. In B.

Bonke, W. Fitch, K. Millar (Eds.), *Memory and awareness in anesthesia* (pp. 131-137). Amsterdam, The Netherlands: Swets and Zeitlinger.

Evans, C., & Richardson, P. H. (1990). A double-blind randomized placebo-controlled study of therapeutic suggestions during general anesthesia. In B. Bonke, W. Fitch, K. Millar (Eds.), *Memory and awareness in anesthesia* (pp. 120-130). Amsterdam, The Netherlands: Swets and Zeitlinger.

Ewin, D. M. (2011). The laws of hypnotic suggestion. In K. Varga (Ed.), *Beyond the words: Communication and suggestion in medical practice* (pp. 75-82). New York, NY: Nova Science Publishers.

Hammond, D. C. (1990). *Hypnotic suggestions and metaphors.* New York, NY: WW Norton & Company.

Jakubovits, E. Janecskó, M., Varga, K., Diószeghy, C. S., & Pénzes, I. (2011). The Efficacy of preoperative suggestions during general anesthesia in the perioperative period. In K. (Eds.) *Beyond the words. Communication and suggestion in medical practice* (pp. 293-303). New York, NY: Nova Science Publishers.

Jensen, M. P. (2008). The Neurophysiology of pain perception and hypnotic analgesia: Implications for clinical practice. *American Journal of Clinical Hypnosis 51,* 123-148.

Kain, Z. N., Mayes, L. C., Caldwell-Andrews, A. A., Karas, D. E., & McClain, B. C. (2006). Preoperative anxiety, postoperative pain, and behavioral recovery in young children undergoing surgery. *Pediatrics, 118,* 651-658.

Kessler, R. (1997). The consequences of individual differences in preparation for surgery and invasive medical procedures. *Hypnos, 24,* 181-192.

Kessler, R., & Dane, J. (1996). Psychological and hypnotic preparation for anesthesia and surgery: An individual differences perspective. *International Journal of Clinical Hypnosis, 44*, 189-207.

Rossi, E. L., & Cheek, D. B. (1988). *Mind-body therapy.* New York, NY: WW Norton & Company.

Schlanger, J., Fritúz, G., & Varga, K. (2013). Therapeutic suggestion helps to cut back on drug intake for mechanically ventilated patients in intensive care unit. *Interventional Medicine and Applied Science, 5*, 145-152.

Szeverényi, C. S., Csernátony, Z., Balogh, Á., & Varga, K. (2013). Examples of positive suggestions given to patients undergoing orthopaedic surgeries. *Interventional Medicine and Applied Science, 5*, 112–115.

Szeverényi, C., Csernátony, Z., Balogh, É., Simon, T., & Varga, K. (2016). Effects of positive suggestions on the need for red blood cell transfusion in orthopedic surgery. *International Journal of Clinical and Experimental Hypnosis, 64*, 404-418.

Szilágyi, A. K., Diószeghy, C., Fritúz, G., Gál, J., & Varga K. (2014). Shortening the length of stay and mechanical ventilation time by using positive suggestions via mp3 players for ventilated patients. *Interventional Medicine and Applied Science, 6*, 3–15.

Szilágyi, A. K., Kekecs, Z., & Varga, K. (2018). Therapeutic suggestions with critically ill in palliative care. *Annals of Palliative Medicine, 7*, 159-169.

Varga, K. (2017). Suggestive techniques without inductions for medical interventions. In M. P. Jensen (Ed.), *The art and practice of hypnotic induction: Favorite methods of master clinicians* (pp. 114-115). Seattle, WA: Denny Creek Press.

Varga, K. (2013.) Suggestive techniques connected to medical interventions. *Interventional Medicine and Applied Science, 5,* 95-100.

Varga, K. (2015). *Communication strategies in medical settings.* Frankfurt am Main, Germany: Peter Lang.

Wise, T. N., Hall, W. A., & Wong, O. (1978). The relationship of cognitive styles and affective status to post-operative analgesic utilization. *Journal of Psychoanalytic Research, 22,* 513-518.

For Further Reading...

Kekecs, Z., & Varga, K. (2013.) Positive suggestion techniques in somatic medicine: A review of the empirical studies. *Interventional Medicine and Applied Science, 5,* 101-111.

Varga, K. (Ed.). (2011). *Beyond the words: Communication and suggestion in medical practice.* New York, NY: Nova Science Publishers.

Appendix

Presented below is a copy of the standardized text as edited by a patient. The words that are ~~crossed out~~ are the words that the patient deleted; the words presented in **bold type** are the words that she added.

* * *

I relax. This is an important surgery. My body and soul can work together with my surgeons. I ~~know that I~~ am in good hands. I trust the ~~hospital~~ ~~clinic~~ and **I trust** the competence of ~~my~~ **its** doctors. I ~~am~~ feel safe and **I am** at peace with myself. I feel that I am taken care of and **I am** ~~well~~ looked after. I give myself over to my healers. I ~~sleep well and~~ rest ~~calmly~~ ~~and~~ ~~pleasantly~~ **comfortably**. Easily and comfortably.

Meanwhile, I see comforting images of my approaching recovery. I can get in touch with and activate my inner capabilities. ~~My inner healing capacity gets stronger and stronger.~~ I am calm and ~~I am~~ at peace with myself. My heart is **calm** and ~~my heartbeat~~ is regular. ~~it is surprising how good I feel...~~ **I feel good**.

During surgery ~~and treatments~~ my body ~~easily~~ adapts to the necessary medical procedures. My **blood** circulation and blood pressure ~~are~~ is **always** appropriate ~~at all times~~. **My body retracts all redundant blood from the operation site. Only the right amount of blood gets to the operation's site, exactly as much as needed to supply the tissues. My body is aware that it is a sterile, clean medical procedure, that it is prepared for and can calmly give itself up to. There is no need for bleeding or infection. My blood circulation and the tension of my muscles are exactly right to promote the progress of the surgical treatment and my healing. My body only allows so much blood to the operation's site that can provide enough nutrition to the tissues and help form a healthy, well closed, nice surface. Excess blood flows to other parts of the body. During the operation only the right amount of blood gets to the tissues. My body automatically knows this, which makes me calm.**

Hearing the sounds and noises of the operation, I feel safe because I know I am taken good care of, and that everybody is working for my safety and well-being. All the sounds and noises during the operation lead to healing, better mobility, to a better quality of life for me. These sounds signal that I can soon start using my abdominal muscles again. This makes me hopeful and fills me with joy. My body happily incorporates the mesh and firmly fixes it, in case the use of the mesh turns out to be necessary,

during the operation. The tissues around the mesh are calm and surround the mesh as if it was a natural organic part of the tissue. They know, that with the help of this material, my abdominal wall recovers and I can move easier and better. My muscles get stronger after the operation making it easier for me to move.

~~At~~ By the end of the ~~surgery~~ operation, ~~I will wake up at the right time with pleasant memories... and relaxed. A feeling that my healing has already started floods my consciousness~~ I am aware that my healing has already begun. As I return to my bed, ~~these~~ this pleasant feeling~~s~~ ~~become~~ gets even stronger. My body soon finds its inner harmony.

~~After the surgery~~ I recover quickly and easily after the operation. The dressing, tubes, infusions, during the first few post-surgery days, are all there to help my perfect recovery. Their reassuring presence promotes my comfort, my fast recovery, my strength and perfect healing. My body gets everything it needs for a fast recovery. I sleep and rest perfectly well on the post-surgery days. ~~During the post-surgery days~~ Every day, I wake up more and more joyful, full of a refreshing, rejuvenating and healing energy.

Even if I sense ~~anything~~ pressure around the area of the operation, it only means that the healing has already begun. It ~~is an indication~~ indicates that I should relax and find a more comfortable position. ~~Over time, and with ease, I become even more comfortable. I completely recover...~~

It helps if I follow the instructions of physiotherapists, doctors, nurses. Any stretching, prickling sensation under the dressing reassures me, because it indicates, that the layers fit together perfectly and they are healing. My body knows how I can fully recover. My blood circulation, immune system, endocrine system, my muscle tone and everything else adjusts to and serves the needs of my body exactly to support perfect healing. They work exactly the way nature intended them to. The area of the operation is healing well and peacefully. It will be perfectly well. It will be perfectly well.

I am surrounded by caring nurses and doctors. Every time I am examined I feel calm and more and more optimistic. After surgery I can rest easily… and I sleep well. I can move more and more easily every day. I perform my usual daily chores with more and more ease.

Every day my movements get easier and easier and I move more and more. Following the instructions of the physiotherapist, I can get out of bed more and more easily, my muscles get stronger and stronger. I notice the different signs of my body, I know when I need more rest and relaxation.

My bodily functions return to normal, I move more and more easily harmoniously and healthily.

Every swallow is a signal to my body that my bowels can work well; my digestion can be healthy, harmonious and calm. And my appetite is better and better, so I am stronger and stronger every day…

The surgical site is healing as well. It will continue to heal, all on its own. It knows what to do to get perfectly well.

The scar will be a proud reminder of what I will have been through. I feel better and better every day; stronger and stronger; and more and more positive. I am patient and happy. I am open to every positive influence that can promote my recovery… and I can protect myself from any negativity. Near and distant acts of kindness and attentiveness give me

~~energy . They multiply the healing power of my body and the efficacy of any treatments I am receiving.~~

I have more and more inner energy. **Every day I feel better and better, stronger and more hopeful. Patient and happy. I am open to all positive influence, that can help my healing and protect me from** ~~any~~ **negativity.**

~~I can find just the right body-soul balance.~~ **I can find my body-soul balance.** ~~I can savor and enjoy the small pleasures of life; a fine piece of clothing, delicious food, a kind smile.~~ **Every day** I feel stronger and healthier **every day**. Stronger and healthier. My recovery is fast and complete. My recovery is fast and complete.

CHAPTER 4

Hypnosis as Anesthesia for Invasive Procedures

Enrico Facco

Enrico Facco is a professor of anesthesiology and intensive care at the Studium Patavinum – Department of Neurosciences, University of Padua, Italy; a specialist in neurology; a teacher at the Franco Granone Institute (Italian Center for Clinical and Experimental Hypnosis, Turin, Italy), and past president of the European Federation for the Advancement of Anesthesia in Dentistry (EFAAD). He has published extensively—over 300 articles in international medical journals, proceedings, and book chapters—on consciousness and its disorders, the neurophysiology of coma, perioperative anxiety, and chronic pain. He is the author of three books (in Italian): Meditation and Hypnosis: Between Neurosciences, Philosophy and Prejudice *(Facco, 2014)*, Near-Death Experiences: Consciousness and Science at the Boundaries between Physics and Metaphysics *(Facco, 2010), and* The Enigma of Consciousness *(Facco, 2018). He is also the co-editor of two books (in Italian):* Non-Ordinary Mental Expressions *(special topic in* Frontiers of Human Neurosciences, 2015) and* Dental Anesthesia and Emergencies *(Facco, 2011). He has been using non-pharmacological techniques* *(including hypnosis and acupuncture) for many years in both research and clinical practice in the management of headaches, chronic pain, anxiety, sedation, and anesthesia. He travels extensively to present his research findings; to teach clinicians effective strategies to successfully assess and manage chronic pain, preoperative anxiety, and dental phobia (with both behavioral and pharmacological techniques) and provide effective hypnotic sedation and analgesia for surgery in medicine and dentistry. The use of hypnosis as anesthesia for invasive procedures described here closely reflects the strategy he uses in his clinical practice, including the strategy to check the patient's ability to develop hypnotic analgesia.*

* * *

It is commonly accepted that hypnosis was introduced by Franz Anton Mesmer in the 18th century, but its roots probably date back much farther, including both Eastern meditation and incubation—a hypnosis-like healing technique used in ancient Greece (Facco, 2014; Facco, 2017).

Hypnosis has been misunderstood and prejudicially rejected since its inception. In the 1800s, when no pharmacological anesthesia was available, hundreds of surgical interventions with hypnosis as the sole anesthetic were successfully performed, but this was not enough to persuade physicians to accept it. For example, James Esdaile, following his report of over 300 major surgical interventions performed under hypnosis (Esdaile, 1846), had to justify himself in response to medical opposition. Later, Theodore Meynert, at a medical congress in 1889, stated that, "Hypnosis is surrounded by a halo of absurdity. Even recoveries do not prove anything" (quoted by Freud, 1889).

The above-mentioned facts show the ostensible incompatibility of hypnosis with the ruling post-Enlightenment and positivist views, prejudicially leading to facts being denied in order to save accepted axioms and theories (Crabtree, 1988; Facco et al., 2015a; Freud, 1889; Hammond, 2008). As a result, following the first interventions with ether anesthesia in 1846, hypnosis was abandoned until the end of the 20th century.

The revival of hypnosis and its use for anesthesia and analgesia may be due to several factors, including:

1. The development of neurosciences, especially the availability of techniques of functional neuroimaging;

2. The birth of the science of consciousness, a huge area of study endowed with deep epistemological implications (Facco et al., 2015a; Facco et al., 2017; Facco, 2018; Zeman, 2001); and

3. The significant development of regional anesthesia and sedation, which helped to view hypnosis as a potentially useful adjuvant.

The therapeutic potential of a patient's subjectivity in clinical practice—neglected by the ruling mechanistic-reductionist stance—is a revolutionary topic. In fact, the *Practice Advisory for Preanesthesia Evaluation*, published by the American Society of Anesthesiologists (2012), does not even mention the words "anxiety" and "fear," neglecting their clinical relevance. On the other hand, perioperative emotional distress has proved to have a strong influence on both suffering and outcome—including postoperative pain, analgesic intake, wound healing, and recovery (Broadbent & Koschwanez, 2012; Ip et al., 2009; Koschwanez et al., 2015; Mavros et al., 2011; Papaioannou et al., 2009; Rosemberg et al., 1994)—making its management a factor of paramount importance. The time is now ripe to recognize the crucial role of consciousness in pathophysiology and therapy and to give patients back their active role in the process of recovery from pain and suffering (Facco et al., 2017).

Hypnosis and Invasive Procedures

A wealth of data on hypnosis in surgery and invasive procedures, including well-designed randomized controlled trials (RCT), is now available, and several reviews and meta-analyses have clearly shown its usefulness (Facco, 2016; Flammer & Bogartz, 2003; Schnur et al., 2008; Tefikow et al., 2013; Wobst, 2007). The results of the available meta-analyses are robust despite the strong lack of homogeneity in the methods of published studies, including:

1. Hypnosis being guided by the hypnotist, self-hypnosis, or tape-recorded hypnosis;

2. Use of hypnosis in preoperative, intraoperative, and/or postoperative phases;

3. Hypnosis in association with local or general anesthesia; and

4. Interventions ranging from minor to major surgery.

The overall results of these RCTs—including a total of about 2000 patients and over 2000 controls—show meaningful, positive effects of hypnosis on perioperative emotional distress, pain, medication consumption, physiological parameters, duration of surgery, wound healing, and outcome. Furthermore, several studies included behavioral techniques such as emotional support and empathic attention as control procedures, showing the superiority of hypnosis with respect to other behavioral techniques.

With respect to hypnosis as the sole anesthesia, only a handful of case studies have been published to date (Botta,

1999; Bowen, 1973; Dias & Ferreira, 1962; Facco et al., 2013; Rausch, 1980; Wain, 2004; Winkelstein & Levinson, 1959). This reflects the above-mentioned rejection of hypnosis until the late 20th century, as well as the safety of modern pharmacological anesthesia and the need for general anesthesia and neuromuscular blocks in most cases. On the other hand, evidence supporting its use as sole anesthesia clearly demonstrates its analgesic power, making it advantageous in the following conditions: (1) minor surgery and minimally invasive procedures, (2) sedation of patients with paradoxical reactions to benzodiazepines, and (3) patients with conditions limiting the use of local and/or general anesthesia. This makes hypnosis superior to pharmacological anesthesia in carefully selected cases, such as for patients with multiple chemical sensitivity (Facco et al., 2013) or for pregnant women with malignancies—for example, thyroid cancer—where a conflict between optimal maternal therapy and fetal well-being exists (Khaled et al., 2016; Mazzaferri, 2011; Oduncu et al., 2003). Here, the uncertainties about the risks imposed by anesthesia may be addressed by hypnosis, either alone or in association with local anesthesia. Hypnotic analgesia can also be used to block the stress reaction, making it possible to keep cardiovascular conditions steady, thus protecting the patient from the surgical "aggression." This protection has been reported both in surgery (Facco et al., 2013) and in experimental studies on pain (Casiglia et al., 2007; Casiglia et al., 2012a; Casiglia et al., 2016).

In short, hypnotic analgesia has been found to be as effective as pharmacological anesthesia in studies comparing the two directly. There is no reason to think that they could not be even more effective when given together. Indeed, in my experience, hypnosis tends to improve all outcomes in the surgical setting, whether or not pharmacological anesthesia was also provided, and it has never made things worse.

As far as minimally invasive procedures are concerned, they can be very distressing and may yield bad outcomes, depending on how uncomfortable or unfriendly the technical environment is, on the patient's view of devices and instruments, on staff behavior, and on the patient's level of fear about the loss of autonomy, potential suffering and pain, and possible complications. When the intervention is performed without respect for the patient's subjective needs, it may result in the development of a post-traumatic stress disorder, a well-known fact in dentistry (Facco et al., 2012). In fact, a close correlation between dental phobia and previous bad experiences in both medicine and dentistry has been reported (Facco et al., 2015b); furthermore, the nocebo effect, which stems from a doctor's inappropriate behavior, may cause hyperalgesia and allodynia, worsen therapy adherence, and decrease overall quality of life (Colloca et al., 2008; Colloca & Miller, 2011).

The beneficial effects of hypnosis have been reported in both children and adults in minor surgery, in dentistry, and in minimally invasive as well as non-invasive but alarming procedures (for example endoscopy, cystourethrography, interventional radiology, biopsy, venipuncture, regional anesthesia, radiotherapy, and both positive-pressure ventilation and MRI; Butler et al., 2005; Cramer et al., 2015; Delord et al., 2013; Facco et al., 2012; Flory et al., 2007; Friday & Kubal, 1990; Hermes et al., 2005; Kiss & Butler, 2011; Liossi et al., 2009; Montgomery et al., 2014; Simon, 1999; Simon & Canonico, 2001).

The goals of hypnosis in invasive procedures are twofold. The first goal is to facilitate full relaxation and anxiolysis. The second goal is to increase the patient's pain threshold as much as possible (and up to the level of full surgical analgesia), according to the patient's ability. The use of hypnosis for sedation is easier than hypnosis for analgesia; most people can successfully be hypnotized to cope with a procedure or intervention with full tranquility. At the same time, their (more or less) increased pain threshold may help to decrease potentially unpleasant sensations during the intervention; using hypnosis as sole anesthesia, however, calls for higher hypnotic ability in the patient.

The outcome of hypnosis may be predicted by checking the patient's hypnotizability and, when needed, by checking analgesic ability in a training session, as described below.

The Assessment of Hypnotizability

People vary widely in their level of trait hypnotizability. Moreover, I have found hypnotizability to be a relevant factor in particular with respect to invasive procedures; a context during which a proper patient performance in terms of intensity and duration is essential for the success of the intervention. Despite being relevant, hypnotizability is rarely tested in clinical reports dealing with invasive procedures.

Hypnotizability can be assessed with several scales. Among the available measures, the Stanford Hypnotic Susceptibility Scale (Weitzenhoffer et al., 1959; Weitzenhoffer et al., 1962) is time consuming (about one hour for administration) and is not suitable for clinical purposes with patients. The Stanford Hypnotic Clinical Scale for adults can be administered in 20-30 minutes, a time that is still not optimal for use in the preoperative setting. The Hypnotic Induction Profile (HIP; Spiegel & Spiegel, 2004) allows the clinician to evaluate hypnotic ability in only 5-10 minutes, making it the most manageable scale in the surgical context. The HIP significantly correlates with both Stanford Scales (Frischholz et al., 1980; Gritzalis et al., 2009; Spiegel et al., 1976), but the HIP appears to be more sensitive to psychological disorders, which can influence the patient's capacity for maintaining the hypnotic state.

As rated by the HIP's 0-10 point Induction Score (IS), about 45%-50% of individuals are classified as having high hypnotizability, 35%-40% are classified in the mid-range of hypnotizability (useful for sedation and other therapeutic purposes, but probably unable to develop a full surgical analgesia), and 15%-20% are low or minimally hypnotizable (Facco et al., 2015c; Spiegel, 1977; Spiegel & Spiegel, 2004; Stern et al., 1978).

No data have been reported in the research literature regarding the compatibility of minimal hypnotic abilities with respect to invasive procedures. Therefore, at this moment one can roughly speculate that only highs (i.e., individuals with an IS ≥ 7.5) may develop a surgical analgesia, while only a subset of lows (i.e., with IS < 3.5) may achieve a satisfactory level of hypnotic relaxation enabling them to face the intervention comfortably.

A potentially relevant parameter provided by the HIP is the decrement profile, which defines subjects with some initial hypnotic ability but losing the focus of attention during the test administration, indicating that their hypnotic state inadvertently ended. Such a profile may be associated with a negative outcome. For example, I observed a fearful patient with this profile who underwent a dental procedure involving multiple teeth extractions; he was able to bear only the first premolar removal, following which the intervention was interrupted. It is worth stressing that the decrement profile in the population has an incidence rate of around only 10%-18%. This profile reflects a low capacity to utilize one's hypnotic resources and to keep the ribbon of concentration, as opposed to not being hypnotizable at all. However, the rate of this profile is higher in individuals with psychopathology, reaching its highest values in individuals with psychiatric diagnoses (Facco et al., 2015c; Spiegel et al., 1976; Spiegel, 1977; Spiegel & Spiegel, 2004).

If these ideas are supported by future research, the routine use of the HIP might help to avoid the use of hypnosis in patients with low hypnotizability as well as unrecognized psychopathology, which may interfere with its beneficial effects. Unfortunately, however, no data are currently available about possible hypnotizability thresholds below which hypnosis for invasive procedures might not be advisable; this is a relevant aspect to be explored by further studies.

Hypnotic Analgesia

Instructions for hypnotic analgesia are relevant both when hypnosis is used as the sole analgesic and when it is used in conjunction with pharmacological anesthesia. It allows for improvement in the patient's tolerance to all potentially unpleasant sensations engendered by venipuncture, local, or regional anesthesia and by painful and non-painful stimuli during the intervention.

It is commonly believed that only hypnotic virtuosos (no more than 15%-20% of the population) may undergo hypnosis as sole anesthesia, but at this point this idea relies only on personal opinions or anecdotal reports. Barber and Mayer (1977) suggested that hypnotic pain control might be a more widespread phenomenon in the population than commonly thought, while other authors have reported that suggestions of analgesia can induce selective—though perhaps not well localized—changes in pain perception even in poorly susceptible subjects (Benhaiem et al., 2001).

A further study has shown that, despite the fact that *highs* and *lows* differ in their response to suggestions, significant analgesia may also be achieved by *lows* (Carli et al., 2008). Therefore, successful hypnotic analgesia does not appear to be associated with the depth of hypnosis attained, suggesting that therapeutic interventions might be tailored to take into account other factors, such as context and motivation (Chaves, 1994). The experience of pain may also be modulated at different levels and via different processes, including attention, memory, and the loop between perception and unconscious processing shaping the features of future experience (Chapman & Nakamura, 1998).

Hypnotic analgesia involves the use of suggestions that target different aspects of a patient's experience (e.g., relaxation, dissociation, distraction, neglect, and instructions for hypnotic focused analgesia or HFA), all of which can influence the level of discomfort experienced by the patient. De Pascalis et al. (1999) reported that *highs* showed significantly higher pain thresholds during dissociative imagery and HFA suggestions, as compared to relaxation only. In another study of 31 healthy subjects, the HFA—obtained by combining suggestions of local anesthesia of the right mandibular arch followed by suggestion of neglect of the same area—yielded a mean increase of right first molar pain threshold of 220%, with respect to baseline value. This value was significantly higher than the one obtained in the contralateral tooth, where HFA was not suggested. Furthermore, 45% of cases developed a full analgesia, marked by a maximal pulp tester stimulation (Facco et al., 2011).

To summarize, the specific instructions to achieve HFA include both (1) suggestions for dissociation and neglect and (2) proper information that enables the patient to avoid the misinterpretation of intraoperative sensations and the loop of negative expectations. Providing both types of suggestions may provide the best results.

The Approach to the Patient

Based on the findings and ideas discussed above, hypnosis can be managed as schematically shown in Figure 1. In elective interventions, the HIP can be administered during the preoperative visit in order to assess the patient's hypnotic ability. In selected cases, the patient's analgesic capacity can be assessed in a further hypnotic session. In an emergency, if hypnotizability cannot be evaluated, a rapid induction can be delivered and then regional and/or pharmacological sedation can be added according to the patient's needs.

Induction Script and Instructions for HFA with Commentary

The following description of a hypnotic session is typical of the one I routinely use for invasive procedures, dental care, and surgery. It consists of several components, including induction, deepening, suggestion of favorite place, instructions for HFA, dissociation, and neglect of the operative field. The components can be used all together to maximize the pain threshold or, in some instances, to achieve full analgesia (according to patient's ability); otherwise, one can select only a subset of the components (e.g., induction plus safe place), when only relaxation is needed in non-painful procedures.

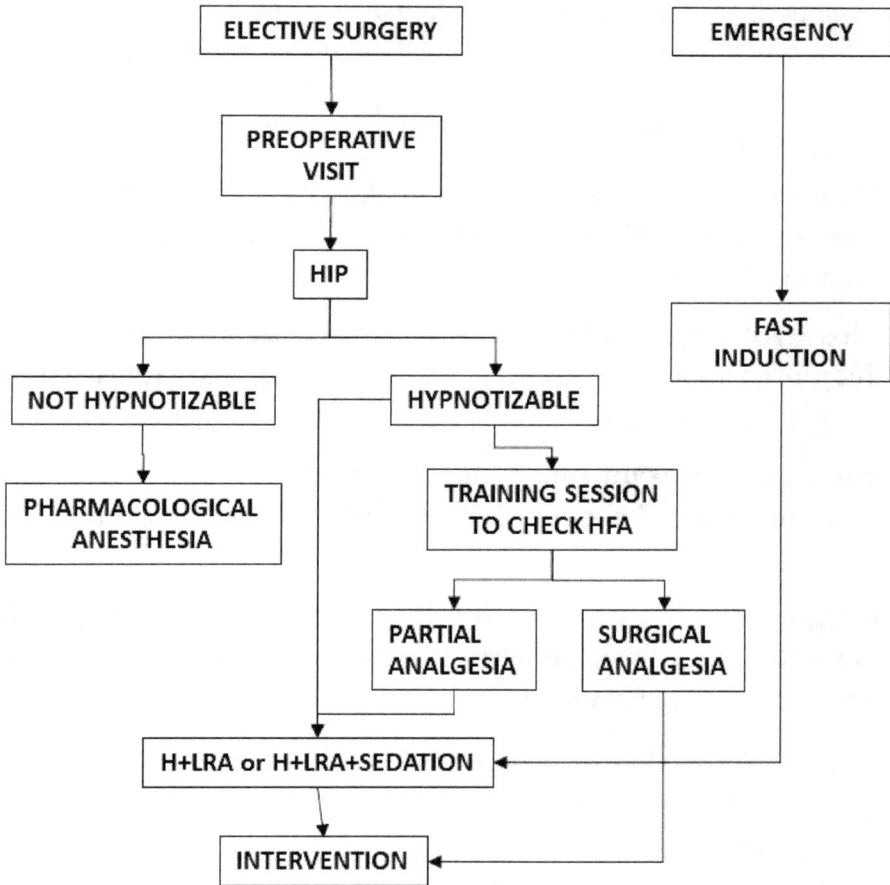

Figure 4.1. The hypnotic approach to the patients for invasive procedures. First, the use of the HIP may help identify patients for whom hypnosis can be successfully used for sedation. Next, according to their hypnotic ability, the intervention can be performed adding local-regional anesthesia (LRA), LRA plus pharmacological sedation, or hypnosis only in selected cases. In an emergency, when there is no time to check hypnotizability, a fast induction can be immediately delivered and, then, the intervention can be performed adding LRA or LRA plus pharmacological sedation, according to the patient's needs.

Induction

[There are many ways to induce hypnosis; each one is suitable, according to the hypnologist's experience. Because I routinely use the HIP prior to hypnotic sessions, I use the same induction, including the Spiegel's eye roll, in the hypnotic session.]

Clinician: Now look towards me. As you hold your head in that position, look up toward your eyebrows—now, toward the top of your head.

Close your eyes, while holding your eyes upward. Take a deep breath, hold. … Now, exhale, let your eyes relax while keeping the lids closed…

You feel a pleasant sensation of relaxation… concentrate on this sensation of progressive relaxation… and let your body float…

Imagine a feeling of floating, floating right down through the bed. There will be something pleasant and welcoming about this sensation of floating.

[The instruction of floating downward instead of upward seems contradictory, but this contradiction of the common expectations concerning the state of floating introduces a paradox, the acceptance of which may be a part of, or will even facilitate the hypnotic experience. Highs may also be inclined to spontaneously "float away" and this paradoxical instruction may help them to refocus their attention.]

And this relaxation spreads to your eyelids, which get heavier and heavier… as if you were going to sleep, a magical sleep… a sleep of someone who is aware he/she is sleeping. … Sliding down inside yourself, into a pleasant, deep, hypnotic trance. … In a cool state of peace…

This relaxed, pleasantly numb feeling is spreading throughout your whole body. ... From your eyelids to your face... neck... arms... legs... your whole body.... You are perfectly relaxed, limp...

Deepening

Deepening may be achieved in different ways, which are not mutually exclusive and may also be combined, according to the preference of the hypnologist. I use one or more of the following.

Awareness of Breathing
(similar to meditation)

Bring your attention to your nostrils... perceive the air flowing towards your lungs... it is fresh. ... An intense and pleasant sensation...

You can also follow the flow of air from your lungs to the nostrils... and realize that the exhaled air is warm and wet. ... It is very different from the inhaled air. ... The inhaled air is rich in oxygen... while the exhaled air is rich in carbon dioxide and water vapor...

When you are breathing, the oxygen reaches your lungs... and then spreads to all the cells of your body... bringing new energy... well-being... relaxation...

[This can be considered as a truism combined with an indirect command. It is undeniable that breathing provides the body with oxygen, and that oxygen is the fuel, while well-being and relaxation are not. However, being that the oxygen-energy relationship is undeniable, it also makes well-being and relaxation a credible, and thus effective, consequence].

Now, if you wish to relax more and more... and reach a state of perfect well-being and bliss... you do not need to do anything special. ... Only let yourself be pleasantly rocked by your own breath... with its unceasing, regular rhythm... like high and ebb tide... and at each respiratory act you will become more and more relaxed... and in a deeper trance... spontaneously... pleasantly... automatically...

Fractionation

Fractionation is an effective way to deepen hypnosis, especially after a rapid induction (Casiglia et al., 2012b; Hammond et al., 1987). It consists of a rapid sequence of induction–dehypnotization–reinduction, exploiting the transient phase of hyper-hypnotizability at the end of a hypnotic session. Fractionation is achieved by instructions for eye-opening without coming out of hypnosis, followed by closing the eyes again, while suggesting that the patient go deeper and deeper each time the eyes are closed; these instructions are usually repeated three to six times.

And now, when I count from 3 to 1, you will open your eyes... but you will remain in a state of hypnosis, deep, hypnosis... and when you close your eyes again, you will relax more and more... you will be a thousand times more relaxed...

3... 2... 1... open your eyes... and now close them again... relaxing more and more...

Safe Place

This instruction is commonly used in hypnosis; it is advisable to ask the patient which places he/she likes, in order to avoid inadvertently bringing them into an adverse, anxiogenic situation (e.g., suggesting a beach or a bath to a subject with a fear of water). The patient may prefer generic places (e.g., beaches, mountains, gardens, etc.) or specific contexts (e.g., I have sometimes been asked for uncommon places, such as Saturnia, a thermal resort in central Italy, or being in the bucentaur [state barge] with the doge during the historical regatta in Venice). The latter calls for some skill to administer and entertain the patient in a scenario the hypnotist may not be familiar with, providing only generic but credible details and letting the patient feel free to imagine what he/she knows and likes. A tropical beach is a scenario appreciated by many patients and the one I most often use; it may also be associated to further instructions to deepen hypnosis and reach the proper hypnotic condition to be maintained throughout the intervention, as follows.

And now, while you are relaxing more and more... listening to my voice... focused on my voice... rocked by your breath... you can move to a terrace of a beautiful resort in a tropical isle... the sea is calm, beautifully clear... turquoise... the sand is white...

There are luxuriant palm trees... and you are in full bliss...

Deepening

In front of you there is a staircase with 10 steps, taking you to the beach... when I count to 10, you will go down step by step... and will enter inside yourself more and more... in a deeper and deeper hypnotic trance... 1... 2... 3... 4... 5... 6... 7... 8... 9... 10... Good!

Now you are in this beautiful place, a sort of earthly paradise... where you can only have pleasant sensations... in a cool bliss...

In front of you there is a comfortable sunbed... and you lie down on it, relaxing more and more, while contemplating this beautiful scenery... and you will remain there, resting and regaining all your energy.

[Include all senses in the suggestions, so that the patient's preferred senses are also included, even if they are not known by the clinician].

Suggestions for Analgesia

HFA can be easily induced by a suggestion of local anesthesia, as follows:

Now I shall administer a local anesthesia... which will make "X" insensitive... totally unresponsive... any kind of sensation will fade away... and then disappear...

[Where X = area to be anesthetized—e.g., mouth, arm, leg, etc. When administering the suggestion of anesthesia, it is useful to scrape the target area with the fingers, in order to alter the sensations coming from that area; this is useful as an indirect command when suggesting the analgesia, as described below.]

Now you can probably feel a different sensation in the anesthetized area with respect to the other side. ... It means that the anesthesia is working... and that part of your body is getting less and less sensitive...

[The sensation yielded by scraping witnesses that something is truly occurring there, making the suggestion of anesthesia more credible. The indirect command sounds like this: "If you feel this sensation, you cannot help but to also feel the upcoming insensitivity.]

Any sensation is fading away and the area is going to be fully anesthetized.

Suggestion for dissociation and neglect

Now that X has become totally anesthetized... no sensation from that area can reach your mind. ... But I also ask your (master)mind to do what he/she is able to do... what it has always been doing since your birth...

Your mind is able to perceive what is of interest and not perceive what is irrelevant... for example, if you pay attention to your nostrils, you can clearly perceive the fresh air you are inhaling... it is an intense and pleasant sensation... but, at the same time, you do not feel the sensation of your relaxed back leaning on the bed. ... It is also intense and welcome... now you can concentrate... to fully feel the sensation of relaxed heaviness coming from your back...

But, at the same time, while feeling these sensations, you do not even realize you are breathing. ... Therefore, perceiving and not perceiving are not different things...

Indeed, they are the same thing. ... Because your mind always does it simultaneously with perfect mastery. ... Perceiving what is of interest and skipping what is irrelevant...

And now I am inviting your (master)mind to let go of all sensations coming from X... because they are irrelevant... they are not of interest to your mind... your mind is now only interested in enjoying this beautiful place in full bliss...

X is fully anesthetized and does not send any sensation to your mind. ... Therefore, you can disregard X... it is as if it does not exist at all. ... Simply let it go...

Even more... now I can remove X and take care of it until the end of this nice experience... in order to allow you to enjoy this state of well-being, full bliss in this beautiful place.

[During the procedure, the verbal contact with the patient can be maintained, according to patient's needs and his/her hypnotizability. More or less frequent contact may be achieved with simple reinforcing sentences such as:]

Very good! I am here with you and everything is ok. ... Go on enjoying this beautiful experience in this nice place.

[Trained highs may be left in their hypnotic state without problems even with less frequent or no reinforcing verbal contact. In this case the silence of the operator may be positively communicated as follows:]

Now you feel so well in this beautiful place that I shall not even disturb you with my voice... so that you can enjoy it to the fullest. ... I shall remain here with you and you will hear from me later.

[At the end of the procedure the patient can be dehypnotized using a reverse sequence of the steps used for induction. Here, two ways are usable according to how the patient has been guided. The first is reversing the eye-roll procedure used for induction, i.e.:]

Now I am going to count backwards. At 3 you will be ready. ... At 2, your eyes will again roll upward with your eyelids closed... and at 1, let them open very slowly. Three, you are

ready. ... Two, with your eyelids closed roll up your eyes...
and 1, let them open slowly.

*[The second sequence can be used when the deepening
through the staircase technique has been used:]*

And now you can get up... and go back to the stairs.... Now
I am going to count from 10 to 0. ... And you will go up step
by step... while your eyelids will get lighter and lighter...
and, when I shall count 1, your eyelids will be so light that
you will be able to open your eyes... 10... 9... 8... 7... 6...
5... 4... 3... 2... 1...

*[In both cases, before counting down, suggestions for
postoperative well-being and analgesia can be administered,
such as:]*

You will remain all day long in perfect well-being. ...
Nothing will disturb you. ... You will feel no pain...
because the anesthesia I did will last all day long...

Or you might only feel small, transient, irrelevant
sensations, which cannot disturb your mind.

References

American Society of Anesthesiologists. (2012). Practice
advisory for preanesthesia evaluation. *Anesthesiology, 116,*
1-17.

Barber, J., & Mayer, D. (1977). Evaluation of the efficacy and
neural mechanism of a hypnotic analgesia procedure in
experimental and clinical dental pain. *Pain, 4,* 41-48.

Benhaiem, J. M., Attal, N., Chauvin, M., Brasseur, L., &
Bouhassira, D. (2001). Local and remote effects of hypnotic
suggestions of analgesia. *Pain, 89,* 167-173.

Botta, S. A. (1999). Self-hypnosis as anesthesia for liposuction
surgery. *American Journal of Clinical Hypnosis, 41,* 299-301.

Bowen, D. E. (1973). Transurethral resection under self-hypnosis. *American Journal of Clinical Hypnosis, 16,* 132-134.

Broadbent, E., & Koschwanez, H. E. (2012). The psychology of wound healing. *Current Opinion in Psychiatry, 25,* 135-140.

Butler, L. D., Symons, B. K., Henderson, S. L., Shortliffe, L. D., & Spiegel, D. (2005). Hypnosis reduces distress and duration of an invasive medical procedure for children. *Pediatrics, 115,* e77-e85.

Carli, G., Suman, A. L., Biasi, G., Marcolongo, R., & Santarcangelo, E. L. (2008). Paradoxical experience of hypnotic analgesia in low hypnotizable fibromyalgic patients. *Archives Italiennes de Biologie, 146,* 75-82.

Casiglia, E., Rempelou, P., Tikhonoff, V., Guidotti, F., Giacomello, M., Lapenta, A. M. ... Facco, E. (2016). Hypnotic general anesthesia vs. hypnotic focused analgesia in preventing pain and its reflex cardiovascular effects. *Athens Journal of Health, 3,* 145-158.

Casiglia, E., Schiavon, L., Tikhonoff, V., Haxhi, N. H., Azzi, M., Rempelou, P. ... Rossi, A. M. (2007). Hypnosis prevents the cardiovascular response to cold pressor test. *American Journal of Clinical Hypnosis, 49,* 255-266.

Casiglia, E., Tikhonoff, V., Giordano, N., Andreatta, E., Regaldo, G., Tosello, M. T. ... Facco, E. (2012a).. *International Journal of Clinical and Experimental Hypnosis, 60,* 241-261.

Casiglia, E., Tikhonoff, V., Giordano, N., Regaldo, G., Facco, E., Marchetti, P. et al. (2012b). Relaxation versus fractionation as hypnotic deepening: Do they differ in physiological changes? *International Journal of Clinical and Experimental Hypnosis, 60,* 338-355.

Chapman, C. R., & Nakamura, Y. (1998). Hypnotic analgesia: A constructivist framework. *International Journal of Clinical and Experimental Hypnosis, 46*, 6-27.

Chaves, J. F. (1994). Recent advances in the application of hypnosis to pain management. *American Journal of Clinical Hypnosis, 37*, 117-129.

Colloca, L., & Miller, F. G. (2011). The nocebo effect and its relevance for clinical practice. *Psychosomatic Medicine, 73*, 598-603.

Colloca, L., Sigaudo, M., & Benedetti, F. (2008). The role of learning in nocebo and placebo effects. *Pain, 136*, 211-218.

Crabtree, A. (1988). *Animal magnetism, early hypnotism, and physical research, 1766-1925*. White Plains, New York: Kraus International Publications.

Cramer, H., Lauche, R., Paul, A., Langhorst, J., Kummel, S., & Dobos, G. J. (2015). Hypnosis in breast cancer care: A systematic review of randomized controlled trials. *Integrative Cancer Therapies, 14*, 5-15.

De Pascalis, V., Magurano, M. R., & Bellusci, A. (1999). Pain perception, somatosensory event-related potentials and skin conductance responses to painful stimuli in high, mid, and low hypnotizable subjects: Effects of differential pain reduction strategies. *Pain, 83*, 499-508.

Delord, V., Khirani, S., Ramirez, A., Joseph, E. L., Gambier, C., Belson, M. et al. (2013). Medical hypnosis as a tool to acclimatize children to noninvasive positive pressure ventilation: A pilot study. *Chest, 144*, 87-91.

Dias, M. M., & Ferreira, J. R. (1962). [Appendectomy under hypnoanesthesia]. *Revista Brasileira De Medicina, 19*, 381-384.

Esdaile, J. (1846). *Mesmerism in India, and its practical applications in surgery and medicine.* London, United Kingdom: Longman, Brown, Green and Longmans.

Facco, E. (2010). *Epserienze di premorte. Scienza e coscienza ai confini tra fisica e metafisica.* Lungavilla, Italy: Altravista.

Facco, E. (2014). *Meditazione e ipnosi tra neuroscienze, filosofia e pregiudizio.* Lungavilla, Italy: Altravista.

Facco, E. (2016). Hypnosis and anesthesia: Back to the future. *Minerva Anestesiol, 82,* 1343-1356.

Facco, E. (2017). Meditation and hypnosis: Two sides of the same coin? *International Journal of Clinical and Experimental Hypnosis, 65,* 169-188.

Facco, E. (2018). *L'enigma della coscienza.* Milano, Italy: Mondadori.

Facco, E., Agrillo, C., & Greyson, B. (2015a). Epistemological implications of near-death experiences and other non-ordinary mental expressions: Moving beyond the concept of altered state of consciousness. *Medical Hypotheses, 85,* 85-93.

Facco, E., Casiglia, E., Masiero, S., Tikhonoff, V., Giacomello, M., & Zanette, G. (2011). Effects of hypnotic focused analgesia on dental pain threshold. *International Journal of Clinical and Experimental Hypnosis, 59,* 454-468.

Facco, E., Gumirato, E., Humphris, G., Stellini, E., Bacci, C., Sivolella, S. ... Zanette, G. (2015b). Modified Dental Anxiety Scale: Validation of the Italian version. *Minerva Stomatologica, 64,* 295-307.

Facco, E., Lucangeli, D., & Tressoldi, P. (2017). On the science of consciousness: Epistemological reflections and clinical implications. *Explore, 13,* 163-180.

Facco, E., Manani, G., & Zanette, G. (2012). The Relevance of hypnosis and behavioural techniques in dentistry. *Contemporary Hypnosis, 29*, 332-351.

Facco, E., Pasquali, S., Zanette, G., & Casiglia, E. (2013). Hypnosis as sole anesthesia for skin tumour removal in a patient with multiple chemical sensitivity. *Anesthesia, 68*, 961-965.

Facco, E., Testoni, I., & Spiegel, D. (2015c). Ipnotizzabilità e Hypnotic Induction Profile. In: E. Casiglia (Ed.), *Ipnosi e altri stati modificati di coscienza* (pp. 271-287). Padova, Italy: CLEUP.

Flammer, E., & Bogartz, W. (2003). On the efficacy of hypnosis: A meta-analytic study. *Contemporary Hypnosis, 20*, 179-197.

Flory, N., Salazar, G. M., & Lang, E. V. (2007). Hypnosis for acute distress management during medical procedures. *International Journal of Clinical and Experimental Hypnosis, 55*, 303-317.

Freud, S. (1889). Referat über Auguste Forel, "Der Hypnotismus". *Wiener Medizinische Wochenschrift, 39*.

Friday, P. J., & Kubal, W. S. (1990). Magnetic resonance imaging: Improved patient tolerance utilizing medical hypnosis. *American Journal of Clinical Hypnosis, 33*, 80-84.

Frischholz, E. J., Tryon, W. W., Fisher, S., Maruffi, B. L., Vellios, A. T., & Spiegel, H. (1980). The relationship between the Hypnotic Induction Profile and the Stanford Hypnotic Susceptibility Scale, Form C: A replication. *American Journal of Clinical Hypnosis, 22*, 185-196.

Gritzalis, N., Oster, M., & Frischholz, E. J. (2009). A concurrent validity study between the Hypnotic Induction Profile (HIP) and the Stanford Hypnotic Clinical Scale for Adults

(SHCS:A) in an inpatient sample: A brief report. *American Journal of Clinical Hypnosis, 52*, 89-93.

Hammond, D. C. (2008). Hypnosis as sole anesthesia for major surgeries: Historical and contemporary perspectives. *American Journal of Clinical Hypnosis, 51*, 101-121.

Hammond, D. C., Haskins-Bartsch, C., McGhee, M., & Grant, C. W., Jr. (1987). The use of fractionation in self-hypnosis. *American Journal of Clinical Hypnosis, 30*, 119-124.

Hermes, D., Truebger, D., Hakim, S. G., & Sieg, P. (2005). Tape recorded hypnosis in oral and maxillofacial surgery— basics and first clinical experience. *Journal of Cranio-Maxillo-Facial Surgery, 33*, 123-129.

Ip, H. Y., Abrishami, A., Peng, P. W., Wong, J., & Chung, F. (2009). Predictors of postoperative pain and analgesic consumption: A qualitative systematic review. *Anesthesiology, 111*, 657-677.

Khaled, H., Al, L. N., & Rashad, N. (2016). A review on thyroid cancer during pregnancy: Multitasking is required. *Journal of Advanced Research, 7*, 565-570.

Kiss, G., & Butler, J. (2011). Hypnosis for cataract surgery in an American Society of Anesthesiologists physical status IV patient. *Anaesthesia and Intensive Care, 39*, 1139-1141.

Koschwanez, H., Vurnek, M., Weinman, J., Tarlton, J., Whiting, C., Amirapu, S. ... Broadbent, E. (2015). Stress-related changes to immune cells in the skin prior to wounding may impair subsequent healing. *Brain, Behavior, and Immunity, 50*, 47-51.

Liossi, C., White, P., & Hatira, P. (2009). A randomized clinical trial of a brief hypnosis intervention to control venepuncture-related pain of paediatric cancer patients. *Pain, 142*, 255-263.

Mavros, M. N., Athanasiou, S., Gkegkes, I. D., Polyzos, K. A., Peppas, G., & Falagas, M. E. (2011). Do psychological variables affect early surgical recovery? *PLoS One, 6,* e20306.

Mazzaferri, E. L. (2011). Approach to the pregnant patient with thyroid cancer. *Journal of Clinical Endocrinology and Metabolism, 96,* 265-272.

Montgomery, G. H., David, D., Kangas, M., Green, S., Sucala, M., Bovbjerg, D. H. ... Schnur, J. B. (2014). Randomized controlled trial of a cognitive-behavioral therapy plus hypnosis intervention to control fatigue in patients undergoing radiotherapy for breast cancer. *Journal of Clinical Oncology, 32,* 557-563.

Oduncu, F. S., Kimmig, R., Hepp, H., & Emmerich, B. (2003). Cancer in pregnancy: Maternal-fetal conflict. *Journal of Cancer Research and Clinical Oncology, 129,* 133-146.

Papaioannou, M., Skapinakis, P., Damigos, D., Mavreas, V., Broumas, G., & Palgimesi, A. (2009). The role of catastrophizing in the prediction of postoperative pain. *Pain Medicine, 10,* 1452-1459.

Rausch, V. (1980). Cholecystectomy with self-hypnosis. *American Journal of Clinical Hypnosis, 22,* 124-129.

Rosemberg, S., Marie, S. K., & Kliemann, S. (1994). Congenital insensitivity to pain with anhidrosis (hereditary sensory and autonomic neuropathy type IV). *Pediatric Neurology., 11,* 50-56.

Schnur, J. B., Kafer, I., Marcus, C., & Montgomery, G. H. (2008). Hypnosis to manage distress related to medical procedures: A meta-analysis. *Contemporary Hypnosis, 25,* 114-128.

Simon, E. P. (1999). Hypnosis using a communication device to increase magnetic resonance imaging tolerance with a claustrophobic patient. *Military Medicine, 164,* 71-72.

Simon, E. P., & Canonico, M. M. (2001). Use of hypnosis in controlling lumbar puncture distress in an adult needle-phobic dementia patient. *International Journal of Clinical and Experimental Hypnosis, 49,* 56-67.

Spiegel, H. (1977). The Hypnotic Induction Profile (HIP): A review of its development. *Annals of the New York Academy of Sciences, 296,* 129-142.

Spiegel, H., Aronson, M., Fleiss, J. L., & Haber, J. (1976). Psychometric analysis of the Hypnotic Induction Profile. *International Journal of Clinical and Experimental Hypnosis, 24,* 300-315.

Spiegel, H., & Spiegel, D. (2004). *Trance & treatment.* Arlington: American Psychiatric Publishing.

Stern, D. B., Spiegel, H., & Nee, J. C. M. (1978). The Hypnotic Induction Profile: Normative observations, reliability and validity. *American Journal of Clinical Hypnosis, 21,* 109-131.

Tefikow, S., Barth, J., Maichrowitz, S., Beelmann, A., Strauss, B., & Rosendahl, J. (2013). Efficacy of hypnosis in adults undergoing surgery or medical procedures: A meta-analysis of randomized controlled trials. *Clinical Psychology Review, 33,* 623-636.

Wain, H. J. (2004). Reflections on hypnotizability and its impact on successful surgical hypnosis: A sole anesthetic for septoplasty. *American Journal of Clinical Hypnosis, 46,* 313-321.

Weitzenhoffer, A. M., Hilgard, E. R., & Kihistrom, J. F. (1959). *Stanford Hypnotic Susceptibility Scale Form A and B.* Stanford, CA: Stanford University Press.

Weitzenhoffer, A. M., Hilgard, E. R., & Kihistrom, J. F. (1962). *Stanford Hypnotic Susceptibility Scale Form C.* Stanford, CA: Stanford University Press.

Winkelstein, L. B., & Levinson, J. (1959). Fulminating pre-eclampsia with cesarean section performed under hypnosis; A case report. *American Journal of Obstetrics and Gynecology, 78,* 420-423.

Wobst, A. H. (2007). Hypnosis and surgery: Past, present, and future. *Anesthesia & Analgesia, 104,* 1199-1208.

Zeman, A. (2001). Consciousness. *Brain, 124,* 1263-1289.

CHAPTER 5

The Exciting Adventure Story: Mutual Storytelling to Capture Attention and Create Emotional Involvement

Lonnie K. Zeltzer

Lonnie K. Zeltzer is a distinguished professor of pediatrics, anesthesiology, psychiatry, and biobehavioral sciences in the David Geffen School of Medicine at the University of California in Los Angeles, USA. She is internationally recognized for her work in developing and evaluating innovative treatments for chronic pain in children and adolescents. Her work has been funded by the National Institutes of Health and other funding agencies, and she has published extensively, with over 450 articles and chapters as well as two books on pain in children.

* * *

While strategies for hypnotic involvement in children and adolescents are based on the same principles as those in adults, there are key differences (Kohen & Olness, 2011). For example, children's developmental maturity needs to be considered. Younger children tend not to close their eyes. They often alternate between attention to their environment and to the imagery, and they may not sit still. During a procedure, they often need to know what is happening and need to be given information, reassurance, and help to return to their imaginative involvement.

For an acute pain experience or a medical/dental procedure, the goal of the clinician is to help the child become so fascinated and involved in the imaginative experience that this involvement can supersede the fear of the procedure and pull attention away from the pain. Additionally, the pace of the child's involvement in the imagery needs to increase at points during the procedure that require maximal distraction from pain or anticipated pain (e.g., the needle about to penetrate the skin).

For younger children, achieving this imaginative involvement often includes mutual storytelling in the present tense (e.g., "What do you see now?"). The focus of the imagery should be something of interest to the child; this can be something familiar, such as a favorite television cartoon or a game that the child loves to play. Or it can be a fantasy, as I will describe later in this chapter.

In mutual storytelling, the clinician often points out things of interest or curiosity, directing the child's attention to the imaginative experience rather than to the environment. The clinician may ask questions along the way, such as pointing out things to notice and to puzzle about. For example, "Do you notice the rabbit that just went behind the tree? I wonder what he is doing there? Let's go look."

Topics should not be too scary, since the goal is to enhance imaginative involvement but not increase anxiety. With younger children, since attention span is shorter than in older children and adolescents, the action needs to be fast-paced and exciting, while involving the child in the unfolding drama of the imaginative experience.

It is noteworthy that many adolescents respond similarly to adults. Adolescents are often comfortable with eyes-closed approaches and with the use of ideomotor finger signaling for communication with the clinician. They also often respond as well as adults do to commonly used inductions, deepening techniques, and suggestions. However, for acute pain and pain associated with medical procedures, the topic of the involvement needs to be something that is of interest to the adolescent and often involves imagined action rather than relaxation.

For example, a soccer player may be helped to play the "best game of his career" during the procedure; scoring goals and hearing the crowd "go wild with excitement." The more intense and exciting the action, if it is meaningful to the adolescent, the greater the involvement. Enhanced imaginative involvement is especially important if the intent is to pull the adolescent's attention from the pain or procedure into the imaginative experience. The clinician often can insert cues, such as, "Wow... the ball is coming right to you!"

Within the imaginative involvement, it is helpful to embed a sense of mastery for the child as a metaphor for mastering the feared procedure or anticipated pain. The younger child typically can become immersed almost immediately in the mutual storytelling without any specific "induction procedure." This is typically what happens when stories are read to children.

A child's play activities also typically include imaginative absorption. The child is "driving" his miniature fire engine to put out the fire, or the girl *is* her doll acting out princess scenes or other fantasies. Thus, immersing the child in mutual imagination is similar to playing with the child. It typically involves both the child and the clinician developing a story together, in which parts are enacted in the present tense with support by the clinician for immersion in colors, smells, texture, sounds, and action.

Rather than just telling the child a story with the child acting as a more passive participant, mutual storytelling brings the story alive for the child and includes his or her creativity in shaping the story. Such involvement helps the child feel a sense of control and mastery. It also makes the story the child's story and not the narrator's. For children that require repeated procedures, their sense of mastery improves with each telling of the story, told each time with minor or major variations. It becomes "familiar," as a way of making the entire medical procedure more familiar.

Verbal participation becomes more difficult with dental procedures, where the child's mouth is open and he or she can't comfortably speak. For dental procedures, it is helpful for the clinician to develop the mutual storytelling prior to, and in anticipation of, the procedure so that the story can become "the child's story" and thus familiar.

The clinician (or parent) can then plan with the child to use finger signaling to indicate if the storyteller is moving in the right direction with the story. A plan can be worked out in advance in which one finger is yes and two fingers are no (or finger up is yes, finger down is no, etc.). The narrator can then alter the story based on the child's ideomotor signaling. Practicing this form of mutual storytelling in advance of dental work can be helpful, and can allow the child to feel both familiar with the plan as well as assured that their input will guide the story. For acute post-operative pain, the story can be mutually told in segments over time, allowing the child time to anticipate where the story will lead the next time it is continued.

Adolescents are more likely to be comfortable with ideomotor signaling, and practice in advance of a dental procedure can be reassuring to them. Often, they need a brief induction and deepening, and can then go directly to "the story." However, these rarely involve calm, relaxing images (e.g., of a beach); rather, they more often involve action and mastery.

Adolescents can be encouraged to continue these "self-involved stories" on their own during subsequent procedures, with discussion of the stories at some point after the procedure. Many older children can take the mutual story and in time make it their own, without the need for the clinician's involvement during the dental procedure. It is helpful, though, for the clinician (or parent) to discuss the story after the procedure has been completed. Such retelling of the story helps it "come alive" and sets the stage for self-story mastery for future procedures. The discussion of the story following the procedure also reinforces the child's comfort with his or her ability to master the procedure in this way, and reduces anticipatory anxiety.

Ultimately, the goal over time is to have the child believe that he or she can get through the procedure, not fear the anticipated pain, become calmer and more cooperative during the procedure (making the procedure easier for the clinician to perform), and feel a sense of mastery and control which gets stronger each time. Some children "catch on" rapidly and no longer need the clinician. Some children's parents can be trained to be the other half of the mutual storytelling, rather than the clinician.

A key to mutual storytelling as a hypnotic intervention during acute pain and procedures in children is to closely observe the child's body language, taking cues from those observations. These cues will direct where to go with the story, how calming or exciting it should be in that moment, and when the child needs to check out the environment and be given information and positive reinforcement before going back to the story.

From 1984-89, I spent the summers with the Psychological Medicine Unit at Great Ormond Street Hospital for Children in London. For children who required multiple procedures or who were experiencing acute pain, I asked to be introduced to the child as, "The storytelling doctor from America." This introduction helped the child understand my role, and together the children and I created mutual stories that helped them get through acute post-operative pain and numerous medical procedures.

My initial introduction to hypnosis was in 1975, during my fellowship, when the meeting of the Society for Clinical and Experimental Hypnosis was held in Los Angeles. I attended a workshop on pain and was amazed at how effective imaginative involvement could be to alter pain and other noxious somatic experiences, such as nausea and vomiting. That workshop led to my early research in hypnotherapy for medical procedures and acute distressing somatic symptoms in children (Ellenberg et al., 1980; Kellerman et al., 1983; LeBaron, & Zeltzer, 1984a, 1984b, 1985a, 1985b, 1985c; LeBaron et al., 1988; Zeltzer, 1982; Zeltzer & LeBaron, 1982, 1986; Zeltzer et al., 1979; Zeltzer et al., 1983; Zeltzer et al., 1984; Zeltzer et al., 1991).

Now, many years later, we are learning the many ways that psychological interventions such as hypnotherapy can impact central neural circuits involved in pain (Martucci & Mackey, 2018). We are also learning how repeated acute pain can become chronic central pain (Feizerfan & Sheh, 2015;) as well as more about the neural connectome in general (Kucyi & Davis, 2015). The use of hypnotherapy for acute and procedural pain in children has the potential to alter the development of pain fear, and reduce the likelihood of the chronification of acute pain.

Transcript Illustrating the Exciting Adventure Story Technique with Commentary

What follows is an example of a hypnotic session with an eight-year-old-girl about to have an intravenous line placed (although this could just as easily apply to acute post-operative pain).

Clinician: Today let's go on the adventure we started last time. This time are you Goldilocks or Curlylocks?

Patient: Curlylocks.

Clinician: Great... so Curlylocks and her sister Goldilocks are about to go into the forest with their baskets to pick berries for their mother...

[Bringing a "sister" allows a within-imagery support system; use of a familiar story, at least to start with (Goldilocks and the three bears), allows for a sense of familiarity, given that the hospital or clinic environment is not cozy and familiar.]

Goldilocks and Curlylocks are walking in the forest hearing the beautiful sounds of friendly birds and looking at all the beautiful flowers and smelling these wonderful flowers... the sun is shining through the trees and feeling warm on their shoulders... when suddenly what do they see?

[This allows the child to fully immerse in the imagery with curiosity and participation in the story development. At this point, the child is looking, and, based on our previous version, announces…]

Patient: A path!

Clinician: Right! And what is the path lined with?

Patient: Lollipops!

[Candy (e.g., chocolate kisses) or cookies are very common responses.]

Clinician: Right! And what color are the lollipops?

Patient: Red and yellow and green.

Clinician: Are these regular lollipops or are they Tootsie Pops with a special filling in the center?

Patient: Regular lollipops.

Clinician: Let's walk up the path and, wait, what is up at the end of the path?

[The patient is now getting immersed in the story from our prior session…]

Patient: A gingerbread house!

Clinician: Let's go closer to open the door and see what is inside. Wow! What is the doorknob made of?

Patient: A marshmallow!

Clinician: Is it an ordinary marshmallow or a special marshmallow?

Patient: A special marshmallow… this big!

[Showing me with her hands spread apart.]

Clinician: Can you turn the knob on the door or it is too squishy to turn? What does it feel like when you squeeze it?

Patient: Squishy, but I can turn it.

Clinician: Great. ... Can you turn it and let us go inside the gingerbread house?

[Child becomes involved in turning the imaginary knob with her hand.]

Wow... look inside! What is the floor made of?

Patient: M&M's.

Clinician: What color M&M's do you see?

Patient: Red, brown, yellow, green... oh, and pink ones too! It feels so funny to be walking on a floor made of M&M's.

Clinician: Can you hear them crunch as you step on them? Let's go into the kitchen... I see a table and three chairs. ... What is on the table?

Patient: Three bowls of ice cream!

Clinician: That looks delicious! Let's take a closer look and see what flavors are in the first bowl...

Patient: Vanilla and strawberry.

Clinician: Is there any chocolate sauce or whipped cream?

Patient: Yes. ... There is chocolate sauce AND whipped cream and a cherry on top!

Clinician: Let's peek at the other two bowls of ice cream. What flavors are in the second bowl?

Patient: A banana and chocolate! And marshmallow sauce and M&M's!

Clinician: Wow. ... I can't wait to see what is in the third bowl!

Patient: Peanut butter ice cream and Reese's peanut butter cups and peanut butter sauce and a peanut butter marshmallow on top!

Clinician: Those sound like delicious sundaes! Which ones do you want to taste?

Patient: All of them!

> *[Silence, while she is pretending to take a spoonful of each and smiling after each and saying, "Yummmm!"]*

By this point, the procedure may be over, in which case we will bring this fantasy to a close, in order to, "Save the next episode in the story till next time." Or, at some point during the experience, the child may suddenly notice the nurse with the alcohol rub, in which case I will indicate that the nurse is putting on "the arm" something "nice and cool, like ice cream. ... What flavor ice cream should the nurse put on the arm?"

The child may go back and forth between noticing the nurse and the needle and re-engagement in the fantasy, following brief information and reassurance. At the point of the needle stick, it can be helpful to have some huge, unexpected surprise happen in the fantasy. This will help to pull the child's attention away from the feared needle and to engage the child's curiosity about what is happening in the imaginative experience. Something like:

Clinician: I just heard a loud crash in the other room! Let's go look to see what happened! It looks like Goldilocks tried to sit on a marshmallow chair and squooshed it to the floor! What other chairs are in this room?

Patient: A chair made of chocolate kisses.

Clinician: Are the kisses wrapped in foil or without foil covering them?

Patient: With foil.

Clinician: Let's each pick one and unwrap it and eat it!

The story can continue as long as is needed, with lots of positive reinforcement and praise for being such a "Good explorer!" as a metaphor for being so brave during the needle stick. For children that are highly anxious in general, the mutual storytelling gets the child back home safely. Other children can end the story wherever we end it and can start all over for future pain episodes or procedures.

Typically, the stories involve a sense of mastery for the child who overcomes fears of the unknown (e.g., What is inside the house? Where does the path lead?) and has some control in the destiny of the heroine in the story (i.e., the child). Repetitive stories with new adventures, or, for some children, repeating the same adventure—similar to hearing the same fairy tales over and over—can be helpful when done with the same clinician. Or parents can become the mutual storyteller with their child, with some initial guidance.

Example of a Hypnotic Session with an Adolescent

Here, I present a transcript of a hypnotic session with a 15-year-old who is about to undergo a lumbar puncture.

Clinician: Hi, Eric. Where do you want to go for today's procedure?

Eric: Let's go where we went last time in the spaceship.

Clinician: Great. ... Take a few moments to get comfortable...

[The patient is on the exam table in a sitting, bent-over-forward position for the lumbar puncture.]

And take a few moments to slowly count from 1 to 10... with each breath out getting slower and longer... and noticing that your eyelids might want to close as they may begin to feel heavier... with each higher number until they may feel too heavy to keep open, and if so you can just let them close and feel even more deeply relaxed... knowing that soon you will be taking a special trip in your own spaceship. ... Signal when you are ready to start your trip...

[Eric's finger raises, his eyes are closed, and his breathing is slower.]

Great... let me know when you are at the take-off platform, snugly and safely inside your spacesuit, and ready to climb into the spaceship.

[Eric signals with his finger as in previous sessions where he uses a raised finger to let me know when he is ready for the next suggestion.]

OK... let me know when you have climbed up the steps through the door and into the spaceship, closed the door, and are in the pilot's seat...

[I wait until Eric's finger is raised.]

Before you take off make sure your seat belt is on tight and let me know when you see the steering panel. ... There might be different buttons, levers, or lights but when you find the take-off switch, let me know.

[I wait until Eric's finger is raised.]

As you turn on the engine and start the spaceship, notice the feel of your body securely belted in the pilot's seat and the feel of the spaceship as it starts moving up and up into the sky... noticing clouds that you pass through... even noticing the houses and trees and cars below getting smaller and smaller, until they are so small that they are hard to see...

Let me know when you safely land your spaceship. ... Where are you going today? To the moon or to a planet?

Eric: The moon.

Clinician: Great. So let me know when you land safely on the moon.

[After a while Eric signals with his finger.]

Before you get out of the spaceship, take a few moments to look out the pilot's window and notice all that you see... and the excitement of knowing that you landed your spaceship expertly and gently on the moon's surface. ... Let me know when you have unbuckled your seat belt and opened the spaceship door, lowered the staircase, and are standing at the exit of the spaceship about to go down the stairs to the moon...

[Eric signals with his finger.]

Take a few moments to look around you and notice all the different aspects of the surface of the moon and all that you accomplished, flying so expertly to get here... let me know when you are ready to walk down the stairs onto the surface of the moon.

[After a long while, Eric signals with his finger.]

As you walk down the stairs notice how confident you feel, how in control, as you glide down the stairs feeling relaxed, comfortable, and yet excited to have landed your spaceship so expertly on the moon. ... Let me know when you are down the stairs and on the moon.

[Eric raises his finger after a while.]

Is the moon's air the same as on Earth or lighter or heavier? Do you seem to float in the air, walk on the ground, or move your feet slowly since you feel heavier on the moon than on Earth?

Just take a few moments to notice how this feels as you take a few steps on the surface of the moon. Did you bring your USA flag as you did last time to place into the moon's surface?

[Eric raises a finger.]

Great, so spend a few moments finding a good spot to plant your flag and let me know when you have found it and planted your flag.

[I wait for what seems like a very long while until eventually Eric raises his finger.]

Let me know when you are ready to go back to the spaceship for your journey home.

[Eric raises a finger.]

OK, so let me know when you have climbed back up the stairs, closed the door to the spaceship, and are back in the pilot's seat.

[Finger raised after a bit of time.]

After you put on your seat belt and look at all the buttons, levers, and lights on the dashboard and are ready to start the engine, let me know.

[Eric raises his finger.]

Before you start the engine to take off to return to Earth, take a few moments just sitting there, looking out the pilot's window at the moon's landscape, knowing how expertly you brought your spaceship to the moon. ... Pretty hot stuff!

Ok, signal when you have the engine started and are ready for your return trip to Earth.

[Eric raises his finger.]

Notice the feel and sound of the engine as you start the engine and start the spaceship directed back down to Earth. Notice the stars in the distance and as you get closer you can see the Earth in the distance... even closer as the Earth gets bigger until you find yourself in the clouds gently floating by... until you see the houses, roads, cars, trees below and know that you know exactly where to land your spaceship. Let me know when you have safely landed your spaceship and turned off the engine.

[Eric raises his finger.]

Before you unfasten your seat belt to leave the spaceship, take a few moments to feel what you just accomplished... expertly going to the moon and back... in control, relaxed, and knowing that you can make this special trip whenever you want... each time noticing something new and comforting along the way... whenever you are ready, you can unfasten your seat belt and lower the exit stairs and walk down... looking around you and seeing your family cheering and all of the crowd of people who have come to celebrate your arrival home and cheer your accomplishment!

Take a few moments to just enjoy that feeling of being a celebrity. When you are ready, you can open your eyes by counting back from 10 to 1, noticing how relaxed you feel

and how pleased you are with your accomplishment today, knowing that you can travel to outer space as we did whenever you want to... easily, effortlessly, and with mastery and control.

For an adolescent, it is often disruptive to ask questions that involve verbal answers. It is helpful at the start to ask if the patient would rather signal with a finger or respond verbally to questions. Eric chose to use ideomotor signaling, since he found it less disruptive than talking.

The pacing of the guided imagery is important so that the patient doesn't feel rushed and can have opportunities to truly feel the adventure experience. Often, it may be helpful to suggest sensory experiences such as feeling the cool air on his face or noticing sounds or colors.

Since in this imaginative experience Eric had a spacesuit on, I chose to have him notice what he saw around him. Throughout the imagery I offered comments about how he might feel about himself in accomplishing this special trip, as a metaphor for his mastery of the lumbar puncture.

It should be mentioned that for his second lumber puncture, Eric chose not to have the local anesthetic injection, since he said he didn't need it and it was disruptive to his adventure. Note that my interaction with this adolescent was in the era before conscious sedation and when intravenous anesthetics were used for pain control during lumbar punctures and bone marrow aspirations.

Throughout the experience, I gave Eric opportunities for immersion in the imaginative involvement and provided language that suggested his abilities to master difficult tasks, be in control, and feel good about himself. Bringing his family and others to cheer his arrival home was a metaphor for his feeling good about his family knowing what he just accomplished (i.e., the lumbar puncture) and their feeling proud of him.

References

Ellenberg, L., Kellerman, J., Dash, J., Higgins, G., & Zeltzer, L. K. (1980). Use of hypnosis for multiple symptoms in an adolescent girl with leukemia. *Journal of Adolescent Health Care, 1,* 132-36.

Feizerfan, A., & Sheh, G. (2015). Transition from acute to chronic pain. *BJA Education, 15,* 98-102.

Kellerman J., Zeltzer, L. K., Ellenberg L., & Dash J. (1983). Adolescents with cancer: Hypnosis for the reduction of acute pain and anxiety associated with medical procedures. *Journal of Adolescent Health Care, 4,* 80-85.

Kohen, D. P., & Olness, K. (Eds.). (2011). *Hypnosis and hypnotherapy with children* (4th ed.). New York, NY: Routledge Press.

Kucyi, A., & Davis, K. D. (2015). The dynamic pain connectome. *Trends in Neurosciences, 38,* 86-95.

LeBaron, S., & Zeltzer, L. K. (1984a). Hypnosis and suggestion for the reduction of pain, anxiety, and vomiting in children with cancer. *Kwartaalschrift voor directieve therapie en hypnose* (*The Journal of Directive Therapy in Hypnosis*), 4, 100-109.

LeBaron, S., & Zeltzer, L. K. (1984b). Research on hypnosis in hemophilia: Preliminary success and problems. *International Journal of Clinical and Experiment Hypnosis, 32,* 290-295.

LeBaron, S., & Zeltzer, L. K. (1985a). Hypnosis for hemophiliacs: Methodologic problems and risks. *American Journal of Pediatric Hematology, 7,* 316-318.

LeBaron, S., & Zeltzer, L. K. (1985b). The role of imagery in the treatment of dying children and adolescents. *Journal of Developmental and Behavioral Pediatrics, 6,* 252-258.

LeBaron, S., & Zeltzer, L. K. (1985c). Research on hypnotherapy for the relief of pain, anxiety, nausea and vomiting in children with cancer. *Texas Psychologist, 37,* 12-14.

LeBaron, S., Zeltzer, L. K., & Fanurik, D. (1988). Imaginative involvement and hypnotizability in childhood. *International Journal of Clinical and Experimental Hypnosis, 36,* 284-295.

Martucci, K. T., & Mackey, S.C. (2018). Neuroimaging of pain: Human evidence and clinical relevance of central nervous system processes and modulation. *Anesthesiology, 128,* 1241-1254.

Zeltzer, L. K. (1982). Pilot research explores clinical possibilities of hypnosis: Research review. *NIH Research Resources Reporter, 6,* 1-5.

Zeltzer, L. K., Dash, J., & Holland, J. P. (1979). Hypnotically induced pain control in sickle cell anemia. *Pediatrics, 64,* 533-536.

Zeltzer, L. K., Dolgin, M. J., LeBaron, S., & LeBaron, C. (1991). A randomized, controlled study of behavioral intervention for chemotherapy distress in children with cancer. *Pediatrics, 88,* 34-42.

Zeltzer, L. K., Kellerman, J., Ellenberg, L., & Dash, J. (1983). Hypnosis for reduction of vomiting associated with chemotherapy and disease in adolescents with cancer. *Journal of Adolescent Health Care, 4,* 77-84.

Zeltzer, L. K., & LeBaron, S. (1982). Hypnosis and nonhypnotic techniques for reduction of pain and anxiety during painful procedures in children and adolescents with cancer. *Journal of Pediatrics, 101,* 1032-1035.

Zeltzer, L. K., & LeBaron, S. (1986). Fantasy in children and adolescents with chronic illness. *Journal of Developmental and Behavioral Pediatrics, 7,* 195-198.

Zeltzer, L. K., LeBaron, S., & Zeltzer, P. M. (1984). The effectiveness of behavioral intervention for reducing nausea and vomiting in children and adolescents receiving chemotherapy. *Journal of Clinical Oncology, 2,* 683-690.

For Further Reading...

LeBaron, S., & Zeltzer, L. K. (1996). Children in pain: Evaluation and treatment. In J. Barber (Ed.), *Hypnosis and suggestion in the treatment of pain* (pp. 305-340). New York, NY: WW Norton.

Zeltzer, L. K. (1986). Hypnosis in pain control. In A. Hurtig (Ed.), *Psychological and psychosocial factors in sickle cell disease* (pp. 106-113). Chicago, IL: University of Illinois Press.

Zeltzer, L.K., & LeBaron, S. (1986). The hypnotic treatment of children in pain. In D. Routh & M. Wolraich (Eds.), *Advances in developmental and behavioral pediatrics, Vol. VII* (pp. 197-234). Greenwich, CT: JAI Press Inc.

Zeltzer, L. K., & Zeltzer, P. M. (2016). *Pain in children and young adults: The journey back to normal.* Encino, CA: Shilysca Press.

CHAPTER 6

Communication and Hypnosis During Pregnancy and Childbirth: Little Words, BIG Impact!

Allan M. Cyna

Allan M. Cyna trained in the UK as a general practitioner and then in anesthesiology in the United Kingdom, USA, and Australia. He is currently an anesthesiologist at the Women's and Children's Hospital, Adelaide, and Nepean Hospital, Sydney; clinical associate professor, University of Sydney; director of studies, South Australian Society of Hypnosis; president elect of the Australian Society of Hypnosis; and chair of the Communication in Anesthesia Special Interest Group of the Australian and New Zealand College of Anaesthetists. Dr. Cyna is an author and peer reviewer for the Cochrane collaboration, and his PhD was on the use of hypnosis for pain relief in childbirth. He has published widely on the use of hypnosis and suggestion in the medical setting and is editor-in-chief of the leading book on this topic: Handbook of communication in anesthesia and critical care: A practical guide to exploring the art *(Cyna et al., 2010).*

* * *

**"Whether you think childbirth will be a dreadful or a
fulfilling experience, you are probably right!"
— Adapted from Henry Ford**

Traditionally, the focus of clinicians involved in pregnancy care and childbirth has been on technological and pharmacological advances. However, the value that patients place on communication is frequently underestimated (Fung & Cohen, 2001). Optimizing communication is said to improve health outcomes, increase patient satisfaction, and reduce error, misunderstandings, patient distress, and negligence claims. When any interaction takes place, communication occurs through multiple layers of conscious awareness, making hypnosis highly relevant to this setting. As pregnancy has been shown to increase hypnotizability (Alexander et al., 2009), the use of hypnotic techniques is likely to be a highly effective strategy in pregnancy-related pain management.

Clinicians working with pregnant women are in an ideal position to utilize suggestions, with or without a formal hypnotic induction, to elicit automatic responses that allow potentially painful procedures to be experienced safely and more comfortably across a wide range of situations. These include: (1) the experience of labor contractions and crowning; (2) potentially painful procedures such as intravenous (IV) cannulation; (3) during the conduct of regional analgesia during labor, vaginal birth, and cesarean section; and even (4) for obstetric-related surgical procedures (Wong et al., 2011). Hypnosis can also play an effective role in the management of painful conditions during pregnancy such as pregnancy-related symphysis pubis dysfunction.

After introductions, asking the parturient how she would like to be addressed shows respect and will likely improve rapport. The GREAT (Greeting/Goals, Rapport, Expectations, Addressing concerns, Tacit agreement/Thanks) template can be used to structure and optimize the interaction (Cyna et al.,

2011). The goal of the interaction in the setting of childbirth is invariably how best to ensure the safety and comfort of both mother and baby. Clarifying and validating uncertainty can help avoid misunderstandings and mitigate unrealistic expectations as the interaction progresses. The parturient's wishes regarding analgesia and obstetric interventions will need to be considered and respected, along with the risks and benefits of any proposed procedures for that particular patient.

For many women, this may be their first hospital experience; they may have no model on which to base their interpretation of events. Labor and birth can be so distressing that women frequently are unable to cooperate consciously, despite wanting guidance. Such assistance can be provided in the form of suggestions that allow women to feel in control and to cooperate with their care in a therapeutic way. The latest research in placebo and nocebo (negative suggestions) confirms how communications integrated into clinical practice can be therapeutic, whether communicating with parturients in labor, with midwives or with others (Krauss, 2015).

A Metaphor for Childbirth

The Olympic athlete metaphor allows women to enhance the truisms of physiological change that occur during pregnancy. Pregnancy represents the nine months of training that women undertake when preparing for childbirth. The expectant mother may not know whether she is entering a sprint or a marathon; but whatever the event, she can be reassured that she is fully prepared for any eventuality. This metaphor of an athlete in training allows the woman to feel fully prepared for labor and childbirth. Physiological truisms of pregnancy and childbirth can be incorporated with suggestions of strength and control. Such truisms can include:

1. The central nervous system is adapted for birth—so much so that if you need an anesthetic when pregnant, only two-thirds of the normal dose is required as compared to providing anesthesia to women when no longer pregnant. This is because the progesterone, estrogen, and other pregnancy hormones (such as oxytocin) have enhanced the brain's ability to allow pregnant women to experience contractions as *comfortably as possible*. The daydream thinking that occurs in pregnancy, the so-called "pregnancy brain" facilitates dissociation and out-of-body experiences as labor progresses.

2. Similarly, breathing changes so that women can breathe more effectively during labor.

3. The ligaments and muscles have become soft and elastic, so that as the baby comes down *comfortably* into the pelvis and the perineum "the ligaments can stretch and... stretch and stretch and relax... without you thinking about it... so that there is plenty of room in the pelvis for you to give birth when the time comes. As skin stretches it tends to go numb so that you know that you will have done everything possible to facilitate the safe and comfortable arrival of your baby."

Indeed, every physiological system of the body is undergoing training for childbirth as the baby has been growing, ensuring that at the end of the Olympic event (labor and childbirth), there will be a gold medal (a baby).

Importance of Rapport

For any hypnosis technique to be therapeutic, it is essential to develop patient rapport. Interactions with women in pregnancy can be optimized by the use of explicit or implicit language structures, such as the Listening, Acceptance, Utilization, Reframing, and Suggestion (LAURS) of hypnotic communication (Cyna et al., 2011). Building rapport into everyday clinical practice involves one skill above all others—and that is to *listen*. There are four questions to ask when listening reflectively: First, did you hear what was said? Second, did you understand what was meant? Third, does the patient know that she has been heard? Finally, does the patient know she has been understood?

Determining the answers to these questions requires a "checking-in" process. Rapport is enhanced by listening for meaning and for potential areas for future utilization. Acceptance of where the patient is also enhances rapport and allows for subsequent interactions to be facilitated and optimized. Acceptance is especially useful when there is a conscious-subconscious dichotomy. For example, a women suffering needle phobia who is consciously presenting for treatment, yet subconsciously cannot allow a drip or an epidural to be inserted.

Utilization, for example of a contraction during labor, can frequently be integrated into the induction or as a fractionation for deepening. Contractions can be reframed into positive rather than fearful experiences by suggesting that the meaning of the sensation is that of getting closer to holding the baby (rather than focusing on pain or pain relief). Suggestions can be used to link physiological truisms and develop a yes-set:

The stronger the contraction, the more effective it is... the more effective it is the stronger and more confident you can feel... knowing that you are getting closer to seeing your baby.

Managing Labor Contractions

Descriptions of a contraction that enhances comfort and control can begin by explaining that,

The contractions start gently, they then reach a peak... they last about a minute... and then... there is a rest!

Many women will recognize, or at least are able to begin to imagine, the possibility that this might be achievable. Contractions can also be explained in a meaningful way, as each contraction allows the mother to feel closer to her baby.

The stronger the contraction, the more effective it is... and the stronger you can feel... the more confident you can feel... knowing you are getting closer to holding and seeing your baby for the very first time.

Each time you breathe in during a contraction, you can breathe in its strength and power, and each time you breathe out you can blow away anything unhelpful, any tensions, any discomforts.

Utilizing the Rests Between Labor Contractions

As you know, each contraction is followed by a rest—this is the time to recoup some energy, build up strength, and gain confidence.

Counting breaths silently in the mind during a contraction can be helpful for two reasons. First, it focuses the mother on her breathing, so that with each breath in she can do a silent count. This allows for the suggestion that with each count, she can feel stronger and more in control, and with each breath out she can feel herself blowing away any unwanted feelings, anything unhelpful, any tension or discomfort into the atmosphere. The second thing that counting achieves is that it tells the mother when the rest is coming. For example, if there are eight breaths during a contraction the mother knows that when she reaches the number eight, she will be able to rest. The suggestion can then be given that,

When women focus on the rest, the rest can seem much longer than it really is and the contraction can seem... much shorter than it really is... as the mind drifts into a daydream and moves away from the contractions as they become even more effective.

This also facilitates the mother's focus on a future reality of seeing and holding her baby. Sometimes, the mother forgets to count or finds the contractions too painful to count beyond one or two. If this happens, it is important to reassure the mother that this is quite normal and we can then see if the mother can get beyond the number two with the next contraction. When asked how many breaths she has counted, this can be built upon for the next time there is a contraction. The clinician needs to be aware that as with any focusing technique, this works well with some women but may be unacceptable to others and alternate techniques may be preferred and utilized.

Utilizing Cervical Dilatation

When the cervix (neck of the womb) is 2-3 cm dilated and you are contracting regularly, you are in established labor and are well on the way to *seeing your baby*. At 4-5 cm dilation you are more than half way as you enter the

accelerated phase of the first stage of labor, with the contractions becoming *much more effective.*

The mother can be encouraged to dive beneath the waves of the contractions or to surf over them; or to simply float over them as they increase in intensity and effectiveness.

The stronger the contraction the more effective... and the stronger you can feel, the more confident you can feel, the more in control you can feel. There is nothing you need to try and do, and there is nothing that need bother you as it just seems to happen all on its own. Just trust in the body... the body knows what to do...

Managing the Second Stage

When the cervix is fully dilated this is an exciting time for any mother as she realizes that she can now be an active participant in the birth of her baby.

All the rests that you have had between contractions have allowed you to store more than enough energy to push effectively when the time comes.

This suggestion enhances a sense of control in the second stage (active pushing when the cervix is 10 cm—fully dilated).

LAURS in Acute Situations or in Emergencies

Patient: I can't listen to you. I can't listen to you. I can't listen to you. ... I'm in too much pain!

Clinician: I know you can't listen to me. *[Acceptance]* Even though you can't *listen* [Utilization] you will be able to *hear* [Reframe] everything you need to allow yourself to relax. ... [Suggestion] Every time you breathe in from now on, you will breathe in some strength and control you didn't even know you had... every time you breathe out you will feel

yourself relax. ... There is nothing you need to try and do and nothing else to think about... it will just seem to happen all on its own...

Acceptance of Different Realities

Acceptance is sometimes a difficult concept for clinicians to grasp. There is little point arguing with a patient logically if she is stressed or distressed. Accepting the patient's beliefs or emotions (for a short time) no matter how strange they appear, allows the clinician to build rapport and then move on to a situation that is more therapeutic for the patient. Acceptance may only be required for a few seconds or minutes.

For example, a woman with an intellectual disability was demanding that she go home after she had been anaesthetized with spinal anesthesia. The operating room staff were telling her that she couldn't go home as she was having a cesarean and the patient was getting more and more agitated. However, as soon as the patient was listened to and her "wish to go home" was accepted—

You can go home as soon as you have had your baby and it is safe for you to do so,

—things settled down and the cesarean proceeded uneventfully.

Similarly, a woman in labor was shouting and writhing in the bed exclaiming "I can't count my breaths, it's all too painful." By listening and using the patient's own words, rapid cooperation with the mother's care is frequently possible. For example, the clinician can say,

I know you can't count breaths at the moment *[Acceptance]*, but after this contraction you will find that knowing this will help you to feel more comfortable *[Utilizing the patient's*

own words and suggestion]. **Especially as you know that as you focus on the rest... you can feel more in control as the contractions start to move into the distance** *[Reframe and Suggestion].*

Anger and distress are usually demands for recognition of emotions and, if these are present, the patient may be indirectly telling you that they do not feel that they have been listened to. Where appropriate, the patient's emotions—for example, crying—can be utilized,

It's good to cry—why don't you cry now till you stop? It's nature's way of allowing you to relax.

Reframing

A common communication to women being given antacid before anesthesia for cesarean section is for them to be told to "drink this, it tastes disgusting!" Not surprisingly, the woman frequently grimaces even before drinking the sodium citrate and then states how disgusting it tastes. Interestingly, if one uses the word "horrible" or "salty" the woman will often repeat the word "horrible" or "salty" after an accepted suggestion. If one suggests that the antacid will neutralize the acid in the stomach so that the woman might have a safer anesthetic should she require general anesthesia, there usually is no comment on the taste.

Direct Suggestions

Direct suggestions are readily accepted in labor or during procedures when stress is high.

You will find that... *[or]* **You will be able to...** *[or]* **You may be surprised... how quickly you recover after the cesarean...**

Similarly, after an episiotomy, the clinician can suggest to the patient that,

You can allow yourself to recover more comfortably knowing that the wound is healing and everything is settling down.

Indirect Suggestions

Indirect suggestions take the form of "most" or "some."

Most women find that... once they realize that healing and recovery is occurring... any unwanted sensations can be put to one side while you get on with caring for your baby. [*Or*] **A patient I saw last week found that...**

For example, while I was placing an IV cannula in a laboring woman the patient said, "If you are trying to suggest arm anesthesia I need to tell you that I am a clinical psychologist and am completely unhypnotizable." This communication was utilized and reframed as it was suggested,

That's OK [*Acceptance*]**, the last clinical psychologist that told me that had a complete arm anesthesia in 4.5 seconds.**

The patient's arm immediately became cataleptic and to the patient's surprise (and mine), a 16 G cannula was comfortably inserted. Another example after a vaginal repair or cesarean section, might take the form,

Most people find that they can allow themselves to recover comfortably, knowing that everything is healing and settling down.

Focus on Positive Suggestions

Negative suggestions are ubiquitous in clinical hospital practice, including during childbirth. Although usually given with the best of intentions, such warnings inadvertently produce subconscious responses that adversely affect symptoms or patient behaviors. Negative suggestions such as, "This is going to sting" are commonplace, for example when injecting local anesthetic.

Recent evidence suggests that if such perceptions are described in terms of meaning rather than as a negative experience, pain can decrease. For example, Varelmann and colleagues (2010) investigated 140 pregnant women presenting for regional analgesia who were randomized to receive either (1) the standard suggestion when injecting local anesthetic into the skin of the back, which was "bee sting coming," or (2) told that the "local anesthesia was injected to numb the skin, so that the procedure can be conducted as comfortably as possible." There were markedly increased pain scores in the "bee sting" group, relative to the numbing group (Varelmann et al., 2010).

Similarly, midwives frequently describe crowning of the baby as it is being born as "burning" or the "ring of fire." It would be more helpful to the woman giving birth to reframe it as "numbing as skin stretches" or as an experience or signal that the woman will "...hold your baby very soon."

Positive suggestions such as, "Most people find it is more comfortable than they might have thought" frequently elicit the perception of comfort. On the other hand, telling patients that a procedure "will hurt" increases the likelihood that the perception referred to will be experienced as pain. It may be more helpful to explain why one is performing the procedure, such as local anesthetic infiltration, by saying something like,

"This will numb the skin and allow us to keep you as comfortable as possible while we finish the procedure."

Sometimes there is concern regarding the ethics of not telling patients something will hurt when the clinician thinks that it might. However, the best available evidence suggests that patient (and possibly the clinician's) expectations influence the patient's experience. Thus, it is just as inaccurate to say something "will hurt" as it is to say it "will be comfortable," when there is a possibility that it will "not hurt" or it will "be comfortable."

One may be left wondering what to say when the patient asks, "Will this hurt?" If one responds "No" or "Yes," the chances are that for some patients this will be less than truthful. However, the statement,

Some people tell me it hurts while others are surprised it is a little bit more comfortable than they thought it might be,

is entirely consistent with honesty with the added benefit of giving an indirect positive suggestion that makes the sensation more likely to be interpreted as "comfortable."

Utilizing Physiological Truisms

Functional Residual Capacity (FRC) is the volume of air in the lungs when chest wall muscles are at their most relaxed and intercostals and diaphragm are in balance. Thus, it is a physiological truism when the clinician suggests that,

When you breathe out you will feel yourself relax.

When the patient focuses on breathing as she breathes out to FRC, a subconscious "yes-set" in the brain is set up as chest wall relaxation is subconsciously recognized as maximally relaxed.

When you focus on your breathing, each time you breathe out you will find yourself relaxing even more.

Repetition

Repetition in a variety of forms is one of the most useful ways that suggestions can be reinforced subconsciously. This can be facilitated by using a variety of phrases that mean the same thing. For example, during labor a parturient responding to the suggestion to relax with breathing can then be reinforced by saying, "That's good," "Well done," and/or "That's right," coinciding with the patient's exhalation.

Double Binds

Double binds are statements of comparable alternatives that can facilitate a sense of control by allowing stressed patients the perception of choice when there isn't any. For example, the clinician might say,

When you are *sitting still for your epidural*, would you like to cross your legs on the bed or rest them on a chair?

If the parturient chooses one of these options, she has also indirectly accepted the suggestion that she will (probably) sit still while epidural placement continues.

Failure Words: "Try" and "Not"

"Try" is a failure word and should be used with extreme caution. The word "not" is not heard by the subconscious. This means that when the clinician asks the patient to, "Try not to move" this is a suggestion for the patient to move. This phraseology can be utilized therapeutically for example by asking patients who are saying that they can't relax to, "Try not to relax" as a suggestion to relax (see below).

The Law of Reversed Effect

The Law of Reverse Effect expresses a means of achieving a goal by asking the woman to *try* to do the opposite of what is intended. For example, the anxious patient is asked to,

Try not to relax and it will seem to happen on its own.

The patient consciously will fail "not to relax" but subconsciously the patient will relax as the "not" is ignored by the subconscious.

Using Language Without Jargon

Patients need to understand the suggestions being provided. In this regard, clinician hypnotherapists have a responsibility to communicate in a way that allows the parturient to adequately understand what is being suggested. Unfortunately, this is not always obvious. Research has found that many patients fail to understand one or more terms used by clinicians in the context of childbirth (Babitu & Cyna, 2010).

Checking In

A checking-in process can be used in at least two ways. First, to ensure that both patient and clinician have understood what has been said and meant. Second, as a way for repeatedly getting verbal consent during potentially painful procedures. For example, if the patient is complaining of pain during a procedure, the clinician can ask, "Is it OK to carry on?" and to ask the patient to say "Stop!" if she wishes the procedure to not continue further until she is more comfortable and ready to go on. This checking-in process facilitates a sense of control.

Pregnancy-Related Symphysis Pubis Dysfunction

Following a standard induction and deepening technique, the usual analgesia techniques of arm anesthesia and transfer of anesthesia glove material of the anesthesia glove over the painful site are frequently helpful. We commonly use the "basket of cares and worries," where unwanted perceptions, unnecessary worries, and unhelpful thoughts that are preventing a comfortable and safe birth of the baby can be placed into a container and then allowed to float away with some helium balloons. However, should these techniques be inadequate, a conversation with the subconscious using ideomotor finger signals can be utilized.

Setting up Ideomotor Finger Signals

Clinician: I am going to call the index finger of the left hand the "Yes Finger." I am going to call the middle finger of that hand the "No Finger." Now imagine the word "Yes"… and when you are imagining the word "Yes" allow the "Yes Finger" to lift up and let me know.

[It does not matter at this stage if the finger lift is or is not conscious.]

When you are imagining the word "No," allow the "No Finger" to lift up and let me know.

[Once the middle finger moves the therapist can say,]

Each time you answer a question you will go deeper into hypnosis, so that it is maximally effective for you. At some point, the fingers will just seem to be answering questions all on their own without you doing anything about it. When in that deepest part of your mind, you are as relaxed and comfortable as you can be for just now, the "Yes Finger" can lift up and let me know. I am now going to ask the creative

part of your mind to think of three different ways in which the pain can be managed in a way that no longer bothers you, and when that creative part of the mind has thought of the first way, the "Yes Finger" will seem to lift up all on its own without you doing anything about it.

After the finger lifts, the clinician suggests that there is a second way to manage the pain so it is no longer bothersome. Once ideomotor responses confirm three different ways of mitigating or resolving the pain are available, one can confirm with an ideomotor response whether or not this will be effective when the woman comes out of hypnosis.

Hypnosis for procedural pain during childbirth or surgery postpartum can be highly effective using a "believed in" or "lived in" imagination technique and suggestions for anesthesia (Wong et al., 2011).

Summary

Hypnosis and suggestion should be an integral part of almost every aspect of the care of a woman in pregnancy and childbirth. Hypnosis training is not featured explicitly in obstetric or midwifery training programs; this needs to be rectified. A learnable framework may assist clinicians of the future to communicate effectively when their usual strategies are not working. This will likely have many potential benefits for patients. Hypnosis and suggestion are core clinical skills and should be an essential component of the care of the pregnant woman, as well as an area for further research.

References

Alexander, B., D. Turnbull, D., & Cyna, A. M. (2009). The effect of pregnancy on hypnotizability. *American Journal of Clinical Hypnosis, 52,* 13-22.

Babitu, U. Q., & Cyna, A. M. (2010). Patients' understanding of technical terms used during the pre-anesthetic consultation. *Anesthesia and Intensive Care, 38*, 349-353.

Cyna, A. M., Andrew, M. I., & Tan, S. G. M. (2011). Structures. In A. M. Cyna, M. I. Andrew, S. G. M. Tan, & A. F. Smith (Eds.), *Handbook of communication in anesthesia and critical care: A practical guide to exploring the art* (pp. 17-29). Oxford, UK: Oxford University Press: Oxford.

Fung. D., & Cohen, M. (2001). What do outpatients value most in their anesthesia care? *Canadian Journal of Anesthesia, 48*, 12-19.

Krauss, B. S. (2015). "This may hurt": Predictions in procedural disclosure may do harm. *The BMJ, 350*, h649.

Varelmann, D., Pancaro, C., Cappiello, E., & Camann, W. (2010). Nocebo-induced hyperalgesia during local anesthetic injection. *Anesthesia & Analgesia, 110*, 868-870.

Wong, L., Cyna, A. M., & Matthews, G. (2011). Rapid hypnosis as an anesthesia adjunct for evacuation of postpartum vulval haematoma. *Australian and New Zealand Journal of Obstetrics and Gynaecology, 51*, 265-267.

For Further reading...

Andrew, M. I., & Cyna, A. M. (2001). The Obstetric patient. In A. M. Cyna, M. I. Andrew, S. G. M. Tan, & A. F. Smith (Eds.), *Handbook of communication in anesthesia and critical care: A practical guide to exploring the art* (pp. 97-110). Oxford, UK: Oxford University Press: Oxford.

Cyna, A. M., Andrew, M. I., & Tan S. (2009). Communication skills for the anaesthetist. *Anesthesia, 64*, 658-665.

Cyna, A. M., & Lang, E.V. (2011). How words hurt. In A. M. Cyna, M. I. Andrew, S. G. M. Tan, & A. F. Smith (Eds.), *Handbook of communication in anesthesia and critical care: A practical guide to exploring the art* (pp. 30-37). Oxford, UK: Oxford University Press: Oxford.

Faymonville, M. E., Laureys, S., Degueldre, C., et al. (2000). Neural mechanisms of antinociceptive effects of hypnosis. *Anesthesiology, 92,* 1257-1267.

CHAPTER 7

Hypnosis for Managing Pain Associated with Cancer and its Treatment

Guy H. Montgomery

Guy H. Montgomery is an associate professor and director of the Center for Behavioral Oncology at the Icahn School of Medicine at Mount Sinai in New York, New York, USA, and is a licensed clinical psychologist. He is internationally recognized for his research on the use of hypnosis to prevent and control symptoms and side effects associated with cancer and its treatment. His research has been funded by the National Institutes of Health and the American Cancer Society. He has published over 100 empirical articles, has an ongoing National Cancer Institute supported program to train health care providers in providing hypnosis and cognitive behavioral therapy to individuals with cancer, and is co-editor of a book on evaluating the effectiveness of psychotherapies: Evidence-based psychotherapy: The state of the science and practice *(David et al., 2017). Dr. Montgomery's work in hypnosis has been recognized through awards he has received, including the Distinguished Contributions to Scientific Hypnosis and Professional Hypnosis Awards from the American Psychological Association's Society of Psychological Hypnosis. For over 20 years, Dr. Montgomery has worked clinically with patients with cancer to help them improve their quality of life, and he continues to be an active clinician in his role as director of psychological services at*

Mount Sinai's Dubin Breast Center. His group has used the hypnosis script presented here to help individuals with cancer to control pain associated with the disease and its treatment. The script includes the approaches and suggestions that have been found, by both patients and providers, to be clinically efficacious, enjoyable, and absorbing.

* * *

Over 15 million Americans are living with cancer today, and nearly two million more are expected to be diagnosed this year (American Cancer Society, 2017). Unfortunately, as patients make their way through the cancer continuum—from diagnosis, through treatment, to survivorship and end of life—they are often dogged by both acute and chronic pain.

The pain can be caused by both the cancer itself as well as by cancer-related treatments, medication regimens, and procedures. For example, cancer diagnostic procedures including breast, prostate, and bone marrow biopsies can be painful; cancer surgery is painful; radiotherapy can cause painful skin toxicity; chemotherapy can cause painful neuropathy; adjuvant medications to reduce the risk of recurrence, such as aromatase inhibitors, can be associated with musculoskeletal pain; and pain can be a grueling part of a metastatic patient's experience at end of life. Beyond being inherently aversive, such pain affects cancer patients' social, functional, and overall quality of life (Bonica, 1985; Swerdlow & Ventafridda, 2012; van den Beuken-van Everdingen et al., 2016).

As a psychologist working in a cancer setting, hypnosis is one of the most commonly used tools in my clinical toolbox. Why? Well, to be quite frank, I am consistently impressed with how hypnosis offers immediate relief in a way that patients find to be relaxing, enjoyable, and often pleasantly surprising. I use hypnosis because it is a wonderful gift to be able to help patients so quickly—often in under 15 minutes—and so profoundly. I use hypnosis because I find it to be eminently adaptable to the complexities of the cancer setting, where I might be called to meet a new patient for the first time and to help them manage anxiety and pain "STAT!" (e.g., before a chemotherapy infusion, before surgery), or where I might be able to deepen and personalize the intervention after seeing someone for weeks. I use hypnosis because as a clinician I find it rewarding to be of service in this way. And like any scientist-practitioner, I use hypnosis because the evidence of research supports its clinical benefits.

Research literature strongly supports the use of hypnosis for pain control both within and outside of the cancer setting (Montgomery et al., 2000; Montgomery, David et al., 2002; Montgomery, Weltz et al., 2002; Montgomery et al., 2007; Montgomery et al., 2013). Hypnosis can address pain directly and can also influence pain indirectly through cognitive (expectancy) and affective (emotional distress) pathways (Montgomery et al., 2010; Schnur et al., 2008). That is, hypnosis interventions can reduce pain by changing patient expectations for pain and by reducing emotional distress. In recognition of these direct and indirect effects, when working with patients to control and reduce pain, I use hypnotic suggestions to accomplish all of these goals.

My first step in delivering a hypnotic pain intervention is to create a relaxing environment (to the extent possible in a busy medical setting). As many practitioners who work in medical settings know, having a dedicated office for psychotherapeutic procedures is often a rare luxury. Just as often, we may be sitting at the bedside, in an infusion suite, in a changing area, a waiting room, or a medical exam room. It can be quite the challenge to make those areas "relaxing," but I always do what I can—closing a curtain, bringing a noise machine, lowering the lights, rolling a stool over to be used as an ottoman, getting an extra blanket to cover a thin gown, etc. I even had a patient ask once to turn the room lights off and just leave the X-ray reader lights on! Whatever makes the patient feel calmer and safer, I accommodate them as much as possible.

Once I have done the best I can with the environment, I next work to develop a strong rapport with the patient. I make sure that we agree on what hypnosis is (and isn't) and that we are on the same page with regard to the tasks and goals of treatment. It is critically important to convey to patients that hypnosis is not magic. If patients have just had an extensive surgical procedure (e.g., a double mastectomy with autologous reconstruction), it is unlikely that they will experience complete pain relief, unless they are *very* hypnotically responsive (i.e., very highly hypnotizable). Surgery is a physical assault on the body, and it is unusual to have the associated pain and discomfort completely disappear. So I convey to patients instead that hypnosis can be used to modulate pain, like turning down the volume on iPhone ear buds.

Second, I explain my rationale for using hypnosis and why I expect it to help reduce their pain. I explain that hypnosis has been used for pain relief for hundreds of years, and has been successful with about every type of pain you can imagine—from headaches to arthritis to surgery to cancer pain. I talk about how efficacious hypnosis is, how quickly it works, and how it has no specific side effects. I define hypnosis based on our published definition (Montgomery et al., 2010), but I do so in terms the patient understands:

Hypnosis is an agreement between a person designated as the hypnotist (e.g., health care professional) and a person designated as the client or patient to participate in a psychotherapeutic technique based on the hypnotist providing suggestions for changes in sensation, perception, cognition, affect, mood, or behavior. (Montgomery et al., 2010, p. 80)

This definition emphasizes three elements that are useful in both setting expectations and reducing emotional distress: (1) Hypnosis is an agreement. Hypnosis is not something that is done to you, rather it is something that we are agreeing upon to do together; (2) Hypnosis is a psychotherapeutic technique intended here to be helpful, restorative, and to relieve uncomfortable sensations. Specifically, in this case we are working to reduce and control your pain; (3) Hypnosis consists of suggestions; not commands or orders but simply suggestions to help you reach your goals.

Third, I move into "debunking," where I work to dispel any myths or misconceptions about hypnosis. Typically, I say:

Before we begin, I have found that it's important to clear up any misconceptions people might have about hypnosis based on things that they might have seen on television or in the movies. [*I usually laugh or smile here to convey that I know how many bizarre/goofy/creepy depictions of hypnosis exist in the entertainment industry. For example, the Oscar-nominated film "Get Out" did not help hypnosis' reputation much...*].

Many people believe things about hypnosis that are not true. These include, first, that hypnosis is something that is done to them rather than something that they can do for themselves; second, that people can lose control of themselves and can be made to do or say anything the hypnotist wants (like cluck like a chicken); third, that they

will feel dramatically different and that they won't be able to come "out" of it when they want to; and, finally, that they won't be able to remember anything about the hypnosis session.

Again, none of these things are true. In fact, hypnosis is something that anyone can do for themselves, and I'm just here to teach you how to do it. Hypnosis is more like focused attention and concentration, so that you can feel more relaxed and comfortable whenever you wish.

Here's one way to think of it. Have you ever been so involved in a book or a show that you lost track of things going on around you? Hypnosis can be like that.

I am asking you to focus on yourself, letting yourself feel more comfortable and relaxed. You will be able to remember everything about this hypnosis session so that you can also use hypnosis on your own, whenever you wish. Today, I am focusing on teaching you how to use hypnosis to better manage your pain. Any questions?

By inviting questions, the hypnosis debunking process opens up a conversation with the patient about hypnosis and its use in cancer care. I make sure to respond to each and every patient question or concern about hypnosis in a reassuring, straightforward, and supportive manner before beginning the formal induction.

For example, a cancer surgical patient might state that, "I am not sure hypnosis will work for me to reduce pain." In order to shape positive expectations while being entirely truthful, I would respond, "I don't know how you in particular will respond, but I do know, based on hypnosis research, that the vast majority of cancer patients benefit from hypnosis." A patient might ask, "Will I lose control during hypnosis?" In order to reduce the patient's distress and fear, I would respond, "You will always be in control, I am just here to guide you."

Fourth, I inquire about the patient's pain, making sure to ask sufficient questions to ensure that I understand their pain experience (e.g., what words or images do they use to describe their pain), so that the suggestions I go on to develop will be empathically accurate. Is the pain sharp, burning, or pulsing? Is it stinging, drilling, or shooting? I use the patient's own language and metaphors when offering suggestions for pain reduction. A mismatch in wording can interfere with patient benefit. For example, if a patient with cancer describes their pain as pulsing, and I suggest that their pain will feel less and less sharp, their expectation for pain relief may be diminished because I have not accurately suggested an improvement in their lived-experience of pain. If my language is not attuned to the patient, at the conclusion of the hypnotic session the patient will likely state the pulsing pain intensity is just as high as it always was. Thus, to ensure benefit and to communicate empathy, I always match suggested reductions in pain with the patient's descriptors of pain.

One general tip for patients with metastatic disease: I actively work to avoid words like "healed" or "healthy." Many patients will find these to be invalidating at best, and distressing at worst, since metastatic generally means incurable. They may never be completely "healthy" again, but they can feel *well, comfortable,* and *at ease.*

As one would expect, many patients with cancer experience heightened emotional distress, particularly around the time of cancer-related medical procedures. Patients undergoing cancer screenings (e.g., biopsy) are justifiably worried about what the tests may find. Surgical patients are often fearful of the procedure itself and the pain that often follows. Chemotherapy patients are often worried about the impact of such an aversive treatment on their whole body. And radiation patients can be concerned about being "burned" by treatment as well as wondering what else the radiation treatments may be doing. As discussed above, as emotional distress often leads to increased pain, I always begin hypnosis sessions with cancer patients with clear instructions, suggestions for relaxation, and suggestions for gradual deepening of a relaxing hypnotic experience.

In order to bring the patient relief from emotional distress in the moment and to promote reductions in pain as the hypnosis session continues, I suggest that hypnotic effects might be "just noticeable" at first—and that the relaxing sensation will then grow, gradually and slowly. From the clinical perspective, this approach helps to avoid failure experiences, which could negate any early, positive expectations about hypnosis. This also helps the patient relax at a time of heightened emotional distress and allows for successes to build—as beginning to feel relaxed reinforces expectations that one will become increasingly relaxed.

In my clinical experience, setting up a "special place" that is relaxing, safe, pleasant, and beautiful contributes to the relaxing experience for individuals with cancer. I state to patients that the place can be real or imagined, and I ask them where they would like to imagine. I leave the choice to patients for two reasons. First, I have found that while a plurality of patients choose a beach scene, it is not a majority. Patients select a wide range of real and imagined places, and I tailor my hypnosis session to their selections. Working in New York City, I've had patients who are more comfortable with the idea of imagining hearing traffic noise from a balcony overlooking Fifth Avenue, or with the peaceful silence of St. Patrick's Cathedral, than with anything associated with nature. I've had patients who chose a scene from the past—a childhood home, a dog who had passed away but was fondly remembered—as well as those who like to imagine the future (e.g., imagining their hair regrown after chemotherapy ends). I let patients be the screenwriter and the director of their own scene. From the clinical perspective, this approach makes for a more positive hypnotic experience and places control of the content of the hypnosis session in the patients' hands. I often catch patients smiling as they enjoy imagining their special place.

Second, this approach allows me to avoid imagery that could be unintentionally triggering for patients. Eliciting patient preferences can avoid patients' fears (e.g., avoid a beach image with a patient who can't swim, has a fear of drowning, or presently has burnt skin due to radiotherapy), avoid triggering unwanted thoughts of death (e.g., floating through the clouds could be understood as a reference to heaven), and avoid triggering thoughts of past trauma (e.g., sexual abuse survivors tend to feel anxious or mistrustful of imagery that suggests a loss of control such as, "your body feels so heavy it feels difficult to move even if you try"). Overall, I find it useful to let patients take the lead.

As the hypnosis session continues and I move into offering suggestions for hypnotic pain relief, I make sure that I do not oversell and suggest that the cancer patient will have no pain. At the same time, I also do not undersell and fail to suggest any pain relief. I want my suggestions to be in the middle of these extremes. I want the patient to have successful experiences of the suggestions for reduced pain, and I want to suggest that their pain relief will grow over time.

Essentially, I am always suggesting pain relief that will grow, then letting the patient experience of pain relief be interpreted as the "correct" response. I work to suggest that there are no wrong experiences. For example, I like to suggest that patients might notice even more pain relief now, or a bit later. In either case, I am setting the expectation of pain relief, without setting up suggestions that are at odds with their experience in the moment.

Individuals with cancer can have flare-ups of their pain at any time. It is not uncommon for postsurgical patients, or patients experiencing bone metastases, to have pain at home, in the middle of the night, and far from the clinics in which we work together. For this reason, when working with individuals with cancer, I like to suggest that they can re-enter hypnosis on their own and use their special place as a way to help them cope with spikes in pain (e.g., breakthrough pain).

In my suggestions, I ask them to focus on their special places and to remember them. In this way, they can return to those places whenever they like. From the clinical perspective, I have seen that approach give hope to patients in that they now have a strategy they can employ when they need it the most. They can do something to control their pain, if they wish, that is not dependent on their "friendly neighborhood hypnotist" being available. I tend to ask patients to come up with their own hypnotic "passwords" that allow them to enter hypnosis and to access their special place. If patients have trouble deciding on a password, I simply suggest they use the words, "hypnosis now," to start them on their way.

When wrapping up a hypnosis session focused on cancer-related pain, I always suggest that the patient will experience continued benefit beyond the session; that they will continue to feel relaxed, well, and at ease. For the patient facing pain and cancer, suggestions to experience continued reductions in emotional distress can go a long way towards keeping pain levels reduced as the patient goes about their day. Hypnosis, and suggested relaxation via a special place, provide patients with a welcome distraction from focusing on cancer and associated physical discomforts. Similarly, projecting expectations for continued pain relief into the future can provide the foundation for patients to experience less pain in the future. Confirmation of these suggested expectations is likely to lead to greater pain relief and add to direct effects of hypnosis on pain control.

After completing the session, I always like to check in with patients to see what we can improve upon in the next session. What aspects of the suggested imagery were clear and easy to imagine, which aspects were more difficult? What changes would they like? It is not surprising to hear the common response that patients were so "relaxed and zoned out" that they may not have any suggestions for changes, because they do not remember the details.

Also, because cancer and its treatment can cause such widespread discomfort, I like to check in on practical issues. Was the patient's body positioning comfortable? Did they feel they needed to get up and move at any point? These are the types of issues that can be practically addressed in order to make the hypnosis session as positive an experience as possible.

As a last point, I am often asked how I recommend hypnosis be used in the context of pain medication. I am not a physician, and I leave all pharmacologic decisions to patients and their medical providers. However, anecdotally, I can share that many patients use hypnosis to help manage their pain while waiting for their pain medications to "kick in."

They often find hypnosis to be tremendously useful in bridging the gap between the sensation of pain, and pain relief from their medications.

Below, I present a hypnosis script that my group at Mount Sinai has found to be useful for controlling pain associated with cancer and its treatment. The script provides examples of much of what I have described above, and I hope it will be a useful tool for other clinicians who work with individuals living with cancer pain.

Hypnosis Script

Clinician: Please make yourself comfortable. Close your eyes and let yourself relax. Take a few slow, deep, and even breaths and notice that as you exhale, you can feel yourself becoming more and more comfortable and more and more relaxed. You can continue to relax, as I speak to you... and each time you exhale, you can feel yourself becoming more and more comfortable... more and more relaxed.

Soon you will experience hypnosis, and you are probably wondering what that experience will be like. I want to assure you that no matter how deeply hypnotized you become... you will remain in complete control.

You will stay in control, even when very deeply involved in the experience of hypnosis. I will make suggestions, but it will be up to you to decide whether you want to experience those suggestions.

If you don't like a suggestion that I make, you can choose to ignore it and to not have that experience. But if you want to experience a suggestion, you may find it easier to experience than you ever thought possible. So the choice is always yours, and it's *safe* to enter hypnosis now, as you allow yourself to relax...

As I speak, you can feel yourself becoming more and more relaxed. But no matter how relaxed you become, you will hear my voice, and you will be able to respond to my suggestions. If you become at all uncomfortable, you can readjust your body and make yourself comfortable again, and that won't get in the way of your experience of hypnosis. If you need to speak to me, you will be able to do so easily, without disrupting your hypnotic experience.

Right now, you might want to relax even more, and as you relax, you may feel a slight tingly feeling in your toes... and if you do, it can comfort you because you will know that it is a feeling of relaxation that some people have as they begin to experience hypnosis.

Let your body relax. Just begin to feel a spreading sense of calm... and peace... letting go of all your cares and concerns, let them drift away, like clouds in the wind... dissipating, more and more at peace... more calm... more comfortable and secure... nothing to bother... nothing to disturb... more and more deeply relaxed, as you enter hypnosis... becoming so deeply involved in hypnosis that you can have all of the experiences you want to have... deep enough to experience whatever you want to experience... but only the experiences you want... just your own experiences.

And you can focus your attention on your toes... your right toes... and your left toes. Let your right toes relax... relax completely... and your left toes. ... Letting your toes relax... more and more... more and more relaxed. And let the relaxation spread from your toes into your feet, and let your feet relax. Let them become more and more relaxed... as you feel so calm and at ease. And now pay attention to your ankles and to your calves. I wonder if you can begin to let go... let go and relax as you feel perhaps a comfortable sense of warmth in your ankles or your calves... in your right leg or in your left leg. Just let your legs relax... more and more comfortable... more and more completely relaxed.

And the relaxation can spread into your thighs... your thighs can relax more and more... just letting go. And you can let your pelvis relax... relaxing more and more. Relax your stomach. Let your stomach become completely relaxed. Just let it go loose and limp... loose and limp. Notice how it feels. Can you let it feel completely relaxed?

Can you notice this now or a bit later? And let the relaxation spread upward into your chest. Let all the nerves and muscles in your chest relax completely... relaxed... loose and limp... feel the peace spreading as you feel so at ease... so secure... your body and mind so relaxed and at peace. And now you can let your back relax, and your shoulders. Let yourself feel the relaxation in your back and your shoulders... more and more relaxed... loose and limp... completely relaxed.

Let the relaxation spread through your arms, down into your hands and fingers. Focus on the feelings in your arms and hands. Do your fingers feel more heavy than light or more light than heavy? Focus on your right upper arm... right lower arm... your right hand... and fingers... relaxing completely... more and more relaxed... completely relaxed. And now your left arm... relaxing completely, so relaxed... completely relaxed. I wonder if you can go even deeper now. Deeper and deeper... just as you wish... just as comfortable and as deep as you would like to go.

Would it feel even better to relax the muscles of your neck? Just let go and relax... loose and limp... completely relaxed.

And relax your jaw muscles. Just let them go limp. All the nerves and muscles in your jaw relaxing completely. And relax all the rest of the muscles in your face... your mouth... nose... eyes... eyebrows... eyelids... forehead... all the muscles going loose and limp... loose and limp... completely relaxed... at peace... comfortable... calm and relaxed... completely at ease. Just let any tension just drop away.

[At this point, we tailor the scene to patient preferences. In every scene, we make sure that the descriptions encourage patients to use all five senses. Below are some examples.]

Beach Script

You might like to imagine being somewhere peaceful and relaxing. I like to imagine lying on a quiet beach on a warm sunny day, with a beautiful blue sky and just a few billowy white clouds floating by. You can picture it in your mind's eye. It is almost like you are really there now, enjoying your special place. You can imagine all the things you would see, all the things you would hear, all the things you would feel, all the things you would touch, all the things you would smell, and all the things you would taste.

You can picture a perfect day at the beach. Looking off into the horizon, where the deep greens and blues of the ocean meet the white clouds and the clear blue sky. You can hear the waves crashing against the shore, the seagulls calling in the distance, perhaps your favorite song playing in the background, or just silence. Comforting. Soothing. You can feel the warmth of the sun on your skin... the cool breeze.

You can imagine stepping into the water, letting the waves roll up your legs. You can imagine swimming or being gently rocked by the waves as you float along facing the sky. You can feel any tension being washed away by the water and replaced with a comfortable, healthy, and easy feeling. You can smell the freshness of the salt-sea air, and imagine the taste of a cool drink. It's almost as if you are really there now, enjoying a beautiful day at the beach.

Feeling relaxed, letting the rolling waves soothe you. Take a moment to just be there now. Take a moment, to be at ease and comfortable on a beautiful day at the beach, in your special place.

Mountain Script

You might like to imagine being somewhere peaceful and relaxing. I like to imagine sitting by a beautiful, clear mountain lake, with a beautiful blue sky and just a few billowy white clouds floating over the peaks. You can picture it in your mind's eye. It is almost like you are really there now, enjoying your special place.

You can imagine all the things you would see, all the things you would hear, all the things you would feel, all the things you would touch, all the things you would smell, and all the things you would taste. You can see the perfect blue sky, stretching off into the horizon where the sky meets the snow-capped mountains. You can see a cozy log cabin, with a wisp of smoke rising from the chimney.

There is a rocking chair on the front porch. ... A perfect place to sit, gently rocking back and forth. You can hear the trees rustling in the wind. Like a lullaby. A gentle sound, soft and comforting. Soothing. The trees are filled with the colors of autumn, orange... yellow... crimson.

The clear lake reflects all these colors back to you. You feel the warmth of the sun on your face and the cool mountain breeze against your skin. You can imagine all this as if you're really there now. You can smell the freshness of the mountain air, the scent of pine, and imagine the taste of a warm drink on a brisk day.

It is almost as if you are really there now. Picture, in your mind's eye, a beautiful day in the mountains. Take a moment to just be there now. Take a moment, to be at ease and comfortable in the mountains, at the edge of a lake, in your special place.

Comfortable Bedroom Script

You might like to imagine being somewhere peaceful and relaxing. I like to imagine lying on a soft, plush, comfortable bed, feeling pleasantly relaxed. It is so quiet and comfortable. You can imagine all the things you would see, all the things you would hear, all the things you would feel, all the things you would touch, all the things you would smell, and all the things you would taste.

There is a big, bright, picture window. It looks out on the most beautiful scenery you can imagine... an endless open field, covered with wildflowers and tall grasses. Gently swaying in the breeze. You can look around your room; it is just perfect. A bed with a warm comforter, an inviting rocking chair, a fireplace in the corner. And you might like to imagine what you would feel... the softness of the bed, the cool clean sheets, the warm radiant heat of the fireplace against your skin...

And you might like to imagine what you would hear... the crackling of the fire, the soft whirr of a fan, your favorite music playing in the background, or maybe it is silent and still. ... And you might like to imagine what you would smell... the clean laundry scent of the sheets, the smell of fresh baked cookies and hot chocolate from the other room, fresh flowers. ... It is almost as if you are really there now enjoying your special place.

Picture, in your mind's eye, relaxing in a perfectly comfortable bedroom. Take a moment to just be there now. Take a moment, to be at ease and comfortable, in this perfect bedroom, in your special place.

Cloud Script

You might like to imagine being somewhere peaceful and relaxing. I like to imagine floating on a cloud. It is so quiet and comfortable. You can imagine all the things you would see, all the things you would hear, all the things you would feel, all the things you would touch, all the things you would smell, and all the things you would taste.

You might like to imagine what you would see... perhaps the dreamy sunset colors of the sky... violet and indigo, lavender and lilac... the view of the earth beneath you... maybe a hint of the silver stars and the moon above... all so tranquil. And you might like to imagine what you might feel... a cool breeze against your cheek, or the texture of the cloud itself.

It might be wispy like cotton, or soft and comfortable like a featherbed... so soft that you can wrap the cloud around you, like a down blanket... floating gently along through the sunset sky. You might like to imagine what you would hear... the wind rushing by, birds in the distance, or maybe it is silent... and still.... And you might like to imagine what you would smell... the crisp freshness of the air, maybe with a hint of pine, or the saltiness of the sea.

It is almost as if you are really there now. And you might like to imagine what you would taste; perhaps the cloud is sweet like cotton candy or marshmallow fluff. Picture, in your mind's eye, relaxing and floating comfortably on a cloud. Take a moment, to just be there now. Take a moment, to be comfortable and at ease, floating on a cloud, in your special place.

And while you are in your perfect place, I am going to count from one to ten. And with each count you can drift more and more deeply into hypnosis... more and more able to experience whatever you want to experience.

One... drift... drift deeper... two... more and more centered, and balanced... three... four... deeper and deeper... five... halfway there... six... seven... even deeper than before... so deep that you can experience whatever you wish to experience... eight... nine... ten... very deep now... very deep... completely at one with yourself... completely engrossed.

While you are in this special place, I would like you to experience all the things you would see... all the things you would hear... all the things you would smell... all the things you would touch... all the things you would taste.... Focus on all these sensations; it is almost like you are really there now, enjoying this special place.

More and more comfortable... more and more relaxed... more and more at ease... more and more deeply hypnotized. It is so perfect. With each breath, you can become more and more deeply hypnotized, so deep that you will be able to do whatever you need to do in hypnosis today... deeper and deeper... deep enough to experience anything you wish to experience. You are so focused; it is almost like you are really there now.

[Tailor the following to the pain descriptors used by the patient and the selected scene.]

Imagine yourself at *[Insert patient's preferred imagery]*. Imagine all the details. Think about what it would be like. It's almost like you are really there now, feeling better and better, more and more comfortable.

I would like you now to focus on your special place. Just be there now, and know that you are at peace, calm and relaxed. There is no tension, no anxiety. Concentrate on this feeling, and know that you can take it with you throughout your day. Imagine yourself feeling relaxed and calm throughout all the parts of your day and night.

No stress... just peace, contentment, satisfaction... well-being... and calm. Nothing can disturb your special place if you don't want it to.... You can choose to be calm and at peace, feeling healthy and relaxed... throughout all the parts of your day.

You are so comfortable in your special place that nothing will disturb you. Your body might feel slightly tingly... slightly warm... but always comfortable. All the parts of your body feel so comfortable and at ease.

You are feeling so comfortable that your pain will hardly bother you at all. You might notice a little pain or *[Insert participant's pain descriptor]*, but those will just be minor annoyances. Nothing you can't handle. You will be comfortable and relaxed, hardly noticing any pain at all. It is almost like your special place protects you from these discomforts throughout your day and as you sleep at night.

Just calm sensations... peace and comfort... healthy and at ease...

You are so comfortable in your special place that nothing will disturb you. You might notice feeling a little pain or *[Insert participant's pain descriptor]*, but it won't get in the way of your ability to do what you need to do, and want to do, throughout your day. You will be as comfortable and as active as you'd like to be, hardly noticing any pain at all.

It is almost like your special place is a source of health, comfort, and well-being. ... There will be little or no pain. All the parts of your body will feel calm and comfortable... and at ease...

From now on, it is going to be very easy for you to become hypnotized whenever you want. We are going to establish a cue that will allow you to be hypnotized instantly. From now on, the words, "hypnosis now" will be a signal for you to enter hypnosis. But it will only work when you say these words, either silently to yourself or out loud, and when you want to become hypnotized.

When you want to enter hypnosis and say the words "hypnosis now," you will immediately become deeply engrossed in the hypnotic experience. But it won't happen if someone else says those words. If you hear these words in normal conversation they will have no effect at all. And it won't work if you do not wish to experience hypnosis. But if you say "hypnosis now" and if you are ready to be hypnotized, you will be able to enter hypnosis immediately. This way you will be able to use hypnosis whenever you like. You can use these words at any time to return to your special place, that place of comfort and peace.

I am going to count backward from five, and with each count you are going to become more and more alert and energized. At the count of one, you can open your eyes. At zero, you will be fully alert and wide awake, feeling better than you did when we began. Five... just starting back... four... feeling the energy rushing in... three... feeling healthy, well, and at ease... two... getting ready to open your eyes... one... open your eyes... zero... alert and wide awake.

Acknowledgements

This research was supported in part by a grant from the National Cancer Institute (R25 CA193098). The content is solely the responsibility of the author and does not necessarily represent the official views of the National Institutes of Health. The author would like to thank Dr. Julie B. Schnur for her invaluable contributions to this manuscript.

References

American Cancer Society. (2017). *Cancer facts and figures.* Atlanta, GA: American Cancer Society.

Bonica, J. J. (1985). Treatment of cancer pain: Current status and future needs. In H. L. Fields, F. Dubner, & F. Cervero (Eds.), *Advances in pain research and therapy* (Vol. 9, pp. 589-616). New York, NY: Raven Press.

Montgomery, G. H., Bovbjerg, D. H., Schnur, J. B., David, D., Goldfarb, A., Weltz, C. R., ... Silverstein, J. H. (2007). A randomized clinical trial of a brief hypnosis intervention to control side effects in breast surgery patients. *Journal of the National Cancer Institute, 99,* 1304-1312.

Montgomery, G. H., David, D., Winkel, G., Silverstein, J. H., & Bovbjerg, D. H. (2002). The effectiveness of adjunctive hypnosis with surgical patients: A meta-analysis. *Anesthesia & Analgesia, 94*, 1639-1645.

Montgomery, G. H., DuHamel, K. N., & Redd, W. H. (2000). A meta-analysis of hypnotically induced analgesia: How effective is hypnosis? *International Journal of Clinical and Experimental Hypnosis, 48*, 138-153.

Montgomery, G. H., Hallquist, M. N., Schnur, J. B., David, D., Silverstein, J. H., & Bovbjerg, D. H. (2010). Mediators of a brief hypnosis intervention to control side effects in breast surgery patients: Response expectancies and emotional distress. *Journal of Consulting and Clinical Psychology, 78*, 80-88.

Montgomery, G. H., Schnur, J. B., & Kravits, K. (2013). Hypnosis for cancer care: Over 200 years young. *CA: A Cancer Journal for Clinicians, 63*, 31-44.

Montgomery, G. H., Weltz, C. R., Seltz, M., & Bovbjerg, D. H. (2002). Brief presurgery hypnosis reduces distress and pain in excisional breast biopsy patients. *International Journal of Clinical and Experimental Hypnosis, 50*, 17-32.

Schnur, J. B., Kafer, I., Marcus, C., & Montgomery, G. H. (2008). Hypnosis to manage distress related to medical procedures: A meta-analysis. *Contemporary Hypnosis, 25*, 114-128.

Swerdlow, M., & Ventafridda, V. (Eds.). (2012). *Cancer pain.* Lancaster, United Kingdom: Springer Science & Business Media.

van den Beuken-van Everdingen, M. H., Hochstenbach, L. M., Joosten, E. A., Tjan-Heijnen, V. C., & Janssen, D. J. (2016). Update on prevalence of pain in patients with cancer: Systematic review and meta-analysis. *Journal of Pain and Symptom Management, 51*, 1070-1090.e9.

CHAPTER 8

Three Hypnosis Techniques for Managing Procedural and Acute Pain with Children

Rob Laing

Rob Laing is a senior staff specialist in children's anesthesia at the Women's and Children's Hospital, Adelaide and a senior clinical lecturer at the University of Adelaide in South Australia. In conjunction with his clinical interests, he uses hypnosis and hypnotic communication with most of his patients and teaches these techniques to hypnosis diploma students, medical students, nursing staff and anesthetic trainees. He has found hypnosis to be particularly effective for managing acute pain, chronic pain, and perioperative anxiety. Here he presents three easily used hypnotic techniques for managing procedural discomfort and acute pain. He has a goal that hypnotic communication and simple hypnotic techniques will become standard practice in all aspects of procedural care with children. His current project is developing a web/app-based resource of hypnotically based techniques for parents and children to access prior to hospital admission.

* * *

Children are great subjects for hypnosis. They are naturally curious, have amazing imaginations, and are less inclined towards critical evaluation than adults are. This chapter describes my three favorite techniques for use with managing procedural anxiety and discomfort. The first technique is "lived-in imagination" which accesses many facets of the hypnotic process, often without mentioning hypnosis. It builds rapport, acts as a pattern break, dissociates, distracts, accesses resourceful states, and induces hypnosis to allow other suggestions for use in the perioperative and procedural discomfort setting. The second technique is hypno-anesthesia utilizing imagery from the "lived-in imagination" technique to suggest perceptual change which induces a numb hand. The third technique is "switch wire imagery," which provides a metaphor that allows children to control the circuitry in their body that transmits pain and sensation.

General considerations for pediatric hypnosis are well covered in the standard pediatric hypnosis texts (Kohen, 2011; Lyons, 2015; Sugarman & Wester, 2013; Thomson, 2005). Universal considerations that I have found important when using hypnosis with children are the use of techniques and language appropriate to their age, development, personality, concentration span, and interests. In addition, working with the child's parents is an integral component of the process. An appreciation of the differences between children, young teens, adolescents, and adults is essential. Flexibility, versatility, creativity, and working with what the child presents to you are essential attributes for the pediatric hypnotherapist.

A core concept for hypnosis that I use is the LAURS (Cyna et al., 2011) of hypnosis.

> Listen—attentively and explore appropriately.
> Accept—the child and parent's reality, at least for the moment.
> Utilize—their reality, likes, dislikes, and words.

Reframe—the problems that are presented.
Suggest—suggestions are given both prior to and during hypnosis.

Therapeutic Strategies

Pain and procedural discomfort have many dimensions. Although we focus on three specific techniques in this chapter, all three fall within a therapeutic strategy which encompasses many techniques to manage the presenting problems and associated goals, including: anxiety management, analgesia, ego-strengthening, use of anchor resourceful states, and forward (also known as age) progression.

Anxiety Management Techniques

Anxiety is managed with some of the following techniques:

1. Hypnosis and accessing a safe place, a favorite place, or favorite activity.

    a. With children, relaxation may not be a concept they understand.

    b. Engaging in a favorite activity may be their way of relaxing.

    c. The favorite activity may be physically active or it may be a mental activity such as computer games, drawing, or painting.

2. Muscle relaxation—progressive muscle relaxation has an important place in pain management.

3. Metaphor—eliminating or modulating anxiety, concerns, and worries by blasting them away, floating

them away, attaching helium balloons and floating them away, and so on.

4. Metaphoric stories—are especially useful when introducing hypnosis as you may never need to introduce the concept of hypnosis, relying instead on the hypnotic qualities of stories and the use of metaphor to provide therapeutic suggestions.

5. Breathing techniques—breathing in bubbles of calm and sending them throughout the body, breathing in strength and blowing away tension, slow breathing.

6. Perceptual changes—find the location, shape, color of the anxiety or other symptom and then change it to give it confident, calm, and capable attributes. One classic change is to find the spinning feeling, take it out of the body, and reverse the spin.

Analgesic Techniques

Analgesic techniques include those that dissociate, distract, and modify perception.

1. Lived-in imagination has components of distraction and dissociation—see transcript below.

2. Switch wire technique—using the wiring for the lights in a room as a metaphor for the nerves supplying the body, find the nerves, see their colors, trace them to the brain, and find the switches, then test the switches (see below).

3. Dissociative or distancing suggestions include placing the pain in one part of the body, distancing oneself from the painful part, or moving yourself away from the pain (e.g., lived-in imagination).

4. Pain perception can be modified by direct suggestion of a numb hand, a magic spot, or transfer of numbness from one part of the body to another.

5. Pain perception can also be altered by changing sub-modalities "What color, shape, texture, temperature is the discomfort? What color, shape, texture, temperature is comfortable?"

Ego-Strengthening and Resourceful States

Utilizing past experiences of success and resilience through the use of anchoring techniques and direct suggestions.

Envisage the Future

Utilizing a metaphoric time machine to go forward to a time when the child has recovered or healed.

Favorite Techniques

What follows are two idealized transcripts of hypnotic sessions which demonstrate three techniques. Scripts are never used, but having a plan is a good starting point. The plan is highly adaptable and is based on the child's presentation. Whenever possible, it is best to work with the child's ideas, words, and concepts, which are elicited during the initial assessment and introduction to hypnosis.

Lived-In Imagination and Hypno-Anesthesia

An 8-year-old girl was referred for hypnotherapy to help manage her fear of needles. She required frequent blood tests and was scheduled for a surgical procedure in two weeks. The goals were to provide suggestions to reduce anxiety, to provide resourceful states to use during venipuncture, and to teach her self-hypnosis to be able to access these states following surgery.

Hypnosis was introduced as a method to help her be the "boss of herself" and to manage her response to blood tests. A more detailed explanation was given to her mother during the phone interview. A history of distress with blood tests was obtained.

She was asked what her name was, what she preferred to be called, and if it was OK for me to call her by that name. We talked about her favorite things, games, books, TV shows, and places. Her favorite things were going for a walk in the forest, coloring in coloring books, and drawing.

Throughout the interview, the LAURS framework was used, with the first phase involving listening and accepting. Rapport was achieved during the pre-hypnotic phase by listening, by enquiring about her favorite things, and by using respectful interaction. As rapport was developed; techniques to make the process interesting and fun increased the engagement of child and parents. An offer of a technique to improve self-mastery is very attractive to most children in this situation.

The child was then offered a brief experience of hypnosis to see what it was like. "All you need to do is use your wonderful imagination..." Hypnosis might or might not be mentioned during the introductory phases—it depends on the referral and the expectations of the family. I do not perform a suggestibility test. Rather, the initial hypnotic experience is really a "hypnosis demonstration"; it's fun, it's something different, and it is not challenging to the child or her parents.

Clinician: Close your eyes and hold out your arms, one hand up and the other hand down. Great, now can you balance a heavy book on this hand [*pressing gently on the hand*], and while you carefully balance that heavy book I'm going to tie two helium party balloons on the other wrist like this [*gently stroke the wrist*], now you can picture those big balloons, pulling up on their ribbons, bouncing against each other...

[*This suggestion might be enough to induce hypnosis by itself.*]

And as the balloons pull that hand up, you can notice the book getting heavier and heavier as you are balancing it, as we add another big book and it gets even heavier. And try to keep them balanced as the other arm feels lighter as those two big balloons are lifting it up. ... Open your eyes and look what's happened.

[*Universally, the observation of one hand angled down and the other one angled up is met with a smile. This is a great start as it allows the family to see that something is happening; the child has an interesting experience and going straight back into hypnosis is a form of fractionation. Next, I introduce the balloon induction (Wicks, 2007).*]

Is it OK if we keep going? That's great. You can let the heavy books drift down, that arm can relax on your lap as you notice the balloons pulling up on the other hand. Now, feel what happens if I push down on that hand, that's right; the balloons just bounce up, and if I push down again, the hand bounces back up [*repeating this several times*].

And it's interesting to notice how the hand just bounces up, and as you notice your hand bouncing up, the rest of your body becomes more relaxed and floppy.

[Continuing to push the arm down and watch it automatically bounce up rhythmically.]

And as the body relaxes, the mind can become more relaxed...

And the interesting thing is, that as the mind relaxes, it can be open to suggestions that can help you...

[The arm can be left suspended as you move to the next phase. This induction follows easily from the balloon and book hypnotic demonstration, it provides a kinesthetic and visual experience with suggestions of relaxation and ends with a cataleptic limb, which provides a test of depth; a convincer for the patient and family that something is happening. The cataleptic limb can be used for further suggestions such as glove anesthesia or as another deepener as it drops into the lap. Next, I introduce deepening using lived-in imagination.]

As your arm comes to rest you can take yourself back to that walk in the rainforest you told me about.

Look around and notice the tall trees, the beautiful flowers...

Take a deep breath and smell all the rainforest smells...

Listen for the sounds of insects and birds.

You can look up through the trees and see the rays of light shining through...

And as you see all the sights, you can step right into the forest, and really be there, taking in all the sights, the sounds, the smells...

[Next, I offer the therapeutic suggestions.]

And as you walk along that path, taking deep slow breaths, feeling stronger with each breath in, feeling happy, knowing that you can come back to this path anytime you need...

And as you breathe out you can feel the whole body relax further...

And as you continue down the path you may notice some butterflies, you can realize how effortlessly they fly, as if they have let go of all their worries...

[With children, deepeners are often not required, and when they are required, simply stacking inductions is sufficient. Lived-in imagination deepens or amplifies the hypnotic state. It can also be used as the sole induction very effectively. In fact, this simple technique could be used in 1-2 minutes for all children having a blood test, a wound dressing, or a catheter procedure to reduce distress and prevent future problems.

There are two approaches to working with lived-in imagination—either by building the experience with information provided by the child prior to hypnosis, using their words and experiences, or by using an interactive approach that allows the child to describe what they are experiencing with directed questions to narrow the experience.]

And as you walk along the rainforest path, feeling stronger and safer, that really happy feeling, you can notice how good that feels, how strong you feel, a feeling that you can do anything, you can achieve anything you want to.

And as that feeling builds, you can touch your thumb and index finger together, pressing hard, locking that feeling in, that's great, really lock it in...

[Here, I anchored the experience.]

As you continue to walk, you can see your friends with you, see the smiles on everyone's face, feeling really happy, it just bubbles up, feeling so good...

And you can lock that feeling in your thumb and finger, that's great...

[An anchor stacking technique. Utilizing the resourceful states from lived-in imagination as an anchor to be accessed later. Continuing to anchor more resourceful states. Amplifying the experience with increased energy and happiness in your vocal tone.]

And as you come to a clearing in the forest, you can feel the sunlight shining through a break in the trees and landing on your body, relaxing you even further...

A butterfly lands on your right hand, and you can be aware of a funny tingling, and that tingling can bring a lovely warm feeling, a comfortable feeling and possibly a puffy feeling, and the other hand is quite different...

[Introducing an anesthetic glove.]

And as you are aware of that tingly, warm, puffy feeling of comfort, as if the hand is being put in the most beautiful magical glove, as if it's been covered in that special anesthetic cream that sinks into your hand, through your skin, through the muscles and all the way to the nerves, feeling more and more numb more and more comfortable, and spreading all the way up to your elbow, more and more numb, tingly and comfortable...

Nod your head if you can feel the comfortable numbness...

Is it Ok if we finish the blood test? That's great, you're doing really well...

You can feel the arm become even more numb as the tourniquet goes on...

And even more numb as I wipe away some sensation...

Locking your thumb and finger together and feeling strong and happy...

[Further utilizing the lived-in imagination to develop a suggestion of numbness in the hand and forearm. Gently touching multiple points on the hand gives a tingling feeling. Hypno-anesthesia is achieved by direct suggestion. Taking blood or a similar stimulus tests the depth of hypnosis and the response of the patient.]

Switch Wire Imagery Technique

This second (idealized) transcript is from a hypnotic intervention used with a 10-year-old girl with 40% burns having wound dressings on the ward. The goal of the intervention was to teach self-hypnosis with suggestions to reduce sensation in the burn area, for use during her debridement and dressing changes. Other suggestions to manage anxiety, appetite, and motivation are used routinely in this situation.

This transcript focusses solely on the "switch wire imagery" (Cyna et al., 2007) and assumes that all the other aspects of hypnosis and trance are in place. It could follow an induction using lived-in imagination, the balloon induction, or countless other techniques.

Switch wire imagery works best in young children to early teens but can be used for older teens and adults. The goal is for the subject to use this technique with self-hypnosis.

Clinician: Would it be OK if we find the wires that run through your body?

It's like the wires in your house—you know, the ones that go to the switches and then to the lights, so when you flick the switch the light goes on or off...

Well, you probably know that your body has wires that run all the way from your brain, down your back to your body, to your arms and to your legs.

In fact, there are different sorts of wires in your body that go to the skin for feeling and to the muscles for moving.

Can you close your eyes, look inside, and find those wires? When you find them can you tell me which color wire goes to the muscles in this arm? Green—that's great.

Now, can you find the wires that go to the skin, what color are they? Red—that's great.

Now, can you find the muscle wires, the green ones and trace them all the way back to your brain until you find the switches?

Great—can you check that the switch is on and lift up the left arm, that's right, now can you turn the switch off, and see what happens. The arm flops down. Try and lift it, it just stays there...

OK, can you do the same thing in your other arm, find the wires, then check the switch is on and the arm is working, lift up the arm and then turn it off...

[Test the arms for tone and floppiness.]

That's fantastic, really good.

Now, can you find the wires that go to the skin in your left arm and follow that wire back until you find the switch?

Have you found it? Great. Now turn that switch off.

The sensation in that arm will be gone now. Is it OK if I test it with a pinch?

[Firm pinch on the back of the hand—no response.]

That's great. Can we test the feeling switch in the other hand? Find the feeling wire, now find the switch. That's great, tell me when you have turned it off, great. Can I test it?

OK, you are really good with those switches. You know you can come back and find those switches any time you need to. You can turn off the switch and make your arm numb whenever you need to.

[The metaphor of a house and the wiring to electric lights is used to help the child find the metaphoric switches that control sensation in his arms. The language subtly incorporates embedded commands, dissociation (__the__ arm), and fail words (__try__ and lift the arm). Avoiding emotive or nociceptive words (e.g., needle, pain, etc.) is important to avoid bringing the patient out of their trance. Permission is asked at each step, especially when the cannula is inserted (e.g., "Is it OK if we put the tourniquet on now?").]

Lived-in imagination is a versatile tool that has many uses—it can induce and deepen hypnosis, it distracts and dissociates, it accesses resourceful starts, and it can be used for self-hypnosis. It is useful at any age and can be used without even mentioning hypnosis.

Hypno-anesthesia can be elicited with direct suggestions utilizing one aspect of lived-in imagination. This can allow a segue—for example, from a butterfly landing on the hand to a magic glove and anesthesia to permit venipuncture—and to test and convince the efficacy of hypnosis.

Switch wire imagery used with hypnotic language can provide a valuable tool for patients to access when a discrete area of the body needs to be switched off.

References

Cyna, A. M., Andrew, M. I., & Tan, S. G. M. (2011). Structures. In A. M. Cyna, M. I. Andrew, S. G. M. Tan, & A. F. Smith, (Eds). *Handbook of communication in anesthesia and critical care: A practical guide to exploring the art* (pp. 17-29). Oxford, UK: Oxford University Press.

Cyna, A. M., Tomkins, D., Maddock, T., & Barker, D. (2007). Brief hypnosis for severe needle phobia using switch-wire imagery in a 5-year old. *Pediatric Anesthesia, 17*, 800-804.

Kohen, D. P. (2011). *Hypnosis and hypnotherapy with children* (4th ed.). New York, NY: Routledge.

Lyons, L. (2015). *Using hypnosis with children*. New York, NY: WW Norton & Company.

Sugarman, L. I., & Wester, W. C., II. (Eds.). (2013). *Therapeutic hypnosis with children and adolescents* (2nd ed.). Bancyfelin, UK: Crown House Publishing.

Thomson, L. (2005). *Harry the hypno-potamus metaphorical tales for the treatment of children*. Bancyfelin, UK: Crown House Publishing.

Wicks, G. (2007). *Hypnosis with children* [DVD]. Educational video available in the South Australian Society for Hypnosis library.

CHAPTER 9

Hypnotic Approaches of Milton Erickson for the Treatment of Acute Pain

Roxanna Erickson-Klein

Roxanna Erickson-Klein worked for many years as a registered nurse and is now a licensed professional counselor in private practice in Dallas, Texas. As the seventh of eight children raised by Milton and Elizabeth Erickson, she benefited from a lifetime of training about the power of hypnosis. Interested in pain management from an early age, she worked with her father initially as a subject and later in a more formal capacity as she began to see how his techniques could be applied to patients in medical settings. She is a member of the Board of Directors of the Milton H. Erickson Foundation, and she is an author, lecturer, trainer, and advocate of clinical hypnosis. Roxanna has worked tirelessly to preserve the original works of her father; co-editing The Collected Works of Milton H. Erickson *with Ernest and Kathryn Rossi is a large part of this effort (Rossi et al., 2008a, 2008b, 2008c, 2008d, 2009, 2010a, 2010b, 2010c, 2010d, 2010e, 2014a, 2014b, 2014c, 2014d, 2014e, 2015). Although the collected works volumes represent most of Erickson's publications, the editors sought to make them more available to readers and to continue facilitating the publications of primary works not yet available to students. Concurrent with this formidable task, Roxanna has written about her own ideas and experiences with hypnosis. The work presented here represents how she has taken what she learned from her father and shared that information, encouraging health care providers in many disciplines to use their own creative ideas for the benefit of individuals with pain or other health conditions.*

*   *   *

Pain is uncomfortable, no question about it. It can rob individuals of their energy, strength, time, monetary resources, attention, and sometimes even their dignity and hope. Although we now benefit from an understanding of the mechanisms of pain, we have made decidedly little progress in empowering patients to accept and deal with sensations that accompany conditions of distress. Milton H. Erickson left a legacy of appreciation for the multitude of ways that hypnosis can mitigate discomfort. In this chapter, I take some of the ideas my father wrote about and other ideas learned directly from him to offer information to professionals interested in helping others cope with acute or procedural pain.

The construct of pain management fascinated my father, as it does me. In the years of Dad's practice (1920s-1980) the concept of acute or procedural pain was not viewed as being distinct from chronic pain, as it often is now. His writings do not specify whether a situation was chronic or acute, although contextual information often helps the reader make this distinction. I think of interventions for acute or procedural pain as "getting through the day," whereas I think of interventions for chronic pain as "getting through a lifetime."

The manner in which Erickson practiced was always individualized to a specific patient, addressing circumstances related to the moment of life's journey that presented. He worked in the now, acknowledging that one's expectations, amassed through previous experiences, affect both reactions to the present as well as the trajectory of opportunity for future responses. Successful intervention in the moment builds the subject's repertoire for additional successes, facilitating healthy adaptation to trials on the near or distant horizon.

The utility of a pain signal to alert the individual to potential or actual injury has important survival value. It warns an individual to guard an injured area, to stop exposing the body to danger, or to seek help in caring for damage that has already occurred. Once the commitment to self-care is fully attended to, the value of the signal is diminished—counterproductive even, to comfort and healing. Beginning with an assessment of what needs attention at this moment, the clinician can then adroitly move into an evaluation of what can be done now to facilitate a comfortable stance that will support an injured individual's treatment and follow-up.

Erickson regarded hypnosis as a powerful adjunct to medical care:

> Hypnosis is a state of awareness in which you offer communications with understandings and ideas to a patient then you let them use those ideas and understandings in accord with their own unique repertory of body learnings, their physiological learnings. Once you get them started, they can then proceed to utilize a wealth of other experiences. (Rossi et al., 2010b, page 316)

The predominant way that Erickson taught students and patients alike was through indirect suggestion, often expressed anecdotally, in which he talked about his own personal, family, and professional experiences. His delivery of these communications involved a hypnotic cadence and a laser-like gaze that he kept fixed on the listener. Like his words, his way of maintaining eye contact was often indirect. While he sometimes maintained a steady, penetrating gaze, at other times he seemed to look away from, or beyond, the individual with whom he spoke. His punctuated moments of emphasis stood out in a powerful manner to create energy and direct attention. His ability to capture an experiential connection was so profound that it drew forth a sense of trust and faith in his abilities. His carefully constructed and incisive suggestions, part of an evolving assembly of opportunities for perceptual change, were always strategically designed to instigate and support one's internal capacity to promote healing.

One of many cases written up by Erickson involved a childhood mishap in which my brother took a fall on our back steps. The case was re-published several times and offers Erickson's own discussion and explanations regarding word choice. What is included here is a succinct version of Erickson's salient comments addressing his precise wording and thinking at the time of the intervention. The case described below is found in Rossi et al., 2008c.

> Three-year-old Robert fell down the back stairs, split his lip, and knocked an upper tooth back into the maxilla. He was bleeding profusely and screaming loudly with both pain and fright. His mother and I went to his aid. A single glance at him lying on the ground, screaming, his mouth bleeding profusely and blood spattered on the pavement, confirmed the existence of an emergency requiring prompt and adequate measures.

No effort was made to pick him up. Instead as he paused for breath for fresh screaming, he was told quickly, simply, sympathetically and emphatically, "That hurts awful, Robert. That hurts terrible."

Right then, without any doubt in his mind, my son knew that I knew what I was talking about. ... Then I told Robert "And it will keep on hurting..." The next step for him and me was to declare, as he took another breath "And you really wish it would stop hurting..." we were in full agreement, and he was ratified, even encouraged in this wish. ... With the situation so defined I could then offer a suggestion with some certainty of its acceptance. "Maybe it will stop hurting in a little while, maybe a minute or two..." a suggestion in full accord with his own needs and wishes, and because it was qualified with 'maybe it will,' it was not in contradiction with his own understandings of the situation.

The next procedure with Robert was a recognition of the meaning of injury to Robert himself—pain, loss of blood, body damage, a loss of the wholeness of his normal narcissistic self-esteem, of his sense of physical goodness so vital in human living. Robert knew he was hurt, that he was a damaged person; he could see his blood on the pavement, taste it in his mouth, and see it on his hands. ... Robert's attention was doubly directed to two vital issues of comprehensible importance to him by the simple statement *"That's an awful lot of blood on the pavement. Is it good, red, strong blood? Look carefully Mother and see. I think it is, but I want you to be sure..."* an open and unafraid recognition in another way of values important to Robert. He needed to know that his misfortune was catastrophic in the eyes of others as well as his own, and he needed tangible proof thereof that he himself could appreciate. ... By declaring it to be 'an awful lot of blood,' Robert could again recognize the intelligent and competent appraisal of this situation in accord with his own actually unformulated, but nevertheless real needs. ... His mother and I examined the blood on the pavement, and we both expressed the opinion that it was good, red, strong, blood therefore reassuring him not only on an emotionally comforting basis only, but upon the basis of an instructional, to him, examination of reality... we qualified that favorable opinion that it would be better if we were to examine the blood by looking at it against the white background of the bathroom sink. By this time Robert has ceased crying and his pain and fright were no longer dominant factors. Instead he was interested and absorbed in the important problem of the quality of his blood. (Rossi et al., 2008c, pp. 34-36)

Erickson goes on in his discussion, utilizing Robert's absorption in the examination of the strength of his blood to address the emergent aspects the injury, including swelling, and the medical interventions needed. *"Next came the question of suturing his lip..."* which Erickson initiated by "stating regretfully that he *'would have to have stiches taken in his lip, it was most doubtful if he could have as many stiches as he could count. In fact it looked as if he could not even have ten stitches, and he could count to 20'"* (Rossi et al., 2008c, p. 36).

Erickson went on to incite a sense of competition within Robert regarding the number of stiches his older siblings had had. "Thus the entire situation became transformed into one in which he could share with his older siblings a common experience with a comforting sense of equality and even superiority. In this way he was enabled to face the question of surgery without fear or anxiety, but with the hope of high accomplishment in cooperation with the surgeon and imbued with the desire to do well with the task assigned him—namely *'to be sure to count the stiches...'* No further reassurances were needed, nor was there any need to offer further suggestions regarding freedom from pain" (Rossi et al., 2008c, p. 36).

In his further discussion about the case summarized here, Erickson points out that at no time was Robert given a false statement, nor was he reassured in a manner contradictory to his understandings. "A community of understandings was first established, and then one by one items of vital interest to him and his situation were thoughtfully considered. ... His role in the entire situation was that of an interested participant" (Rossi et al., 2008c, pp. 36-37).

The back entry to our home with the sharp cement step on which Robert had tripped was rearranged to present less of a hazard, but years later Robert remained proud to show off the exact sharp edge that caused the injury. Today my brother still remembers the fall, his feelings of competition with his older siblings, and his own deep absorption in the process of counting the stiches. When asked, he shows his W-shaped scar like a proudly worn, hard-earned badge. Our lifetime as close and much-loved siblings has offered many occasions for me to notice how Robert engages his skill to become absorbed in some interesting element of the moment, a skill that has been useful and effective in helping him to cope effectively with other painful conditions that life has brought him.

This case is globally relevant to acute or procedural pain as it addresses some essential elements—including the need to be completely honest with the patient. Another element is to let the needs of the situation, bolstered by patient strengths, guide discussion. Never indicate that a procedure "won't be painful" when it might be. My own style is to be very direct; for example, I might say, "Of course it will hurt—there will be a needle sticking through your skin." I offer a straightforward, reassuring expression and factual information about what needs attention and what to expect. This generally evokes a response from the patient that I am a trustworthy, reliable source of needed information. I also add my own truths—for example, "We have worked with similar situations before, and there are a multitude of ways that inevitable discomfort can be minimized."

Confronting the reality of the tasks at hand becomes fertile opportunity for engaging the patient as an active participant. As early in the relationship as possible, I begin to assess the patient's own previous experiences with pain management. This discussion reveals their expectations as well as their readiness to actively engage. The unique qualities individuals bring and their recollections of past successes are a rich indicator of what may be useful in the present. One of the elements that I look for is an evaluation of whether the patient will likely respond better by turning towards the pain or turning away from it.

In Robert's case, the interventions started with turning towards his discomfort—fearlessly confronting the injury and becoming an active participant in the process. In contrast, some individuals and situations lend themselves to turning away from the sensation, having already recognized that they are better served with the expertise of other members of the medical team. While the professional assumes responsibilities to assure that needed interventions are attended to, the patient is free to engage in distraction from the sensations. In contrast, some individuals are hesitant to relinquish control and have personalities that serve the situation more effectively by keeping their attention focused on the injury and the procedures and engaged in their own exploration of sensations.

Distraction is a common, effective way of redirecting attention at a time when focus on uncomfortable signals is not useful. Distraction provides a space within which a suggestion can offer new stimulus to serve the larger needs of the subject. I am reminded of a chaplain who was particularly good at calming patients who were in crisis. When I inquired about his technique he offered, "It's simple, I just get the patients to talk about something interesting to them."

When my siblings and I were children, my father would often respond to our discomfort as an opportunity to relax together. Sometimes we read comic books, individually or in parallel. Many times, Dad would announce, "It is a good time for a story." Dad had the ability to construct tales that involved familiar relatives, pets, friends, patients, or imaginary protagonists. All of the eight siblings shared a love for the familiar cast of characters. The stories always began with a hypnotic rhythm, focus of attention, invitation to relax, and feeling that nothing was nearly so important in this moment as to be together and to attend to the story as it evolves. Paced to adapt to the available time and our own depth of absorption, these respites brought about a shared sense of comfort and relaxation. The characters involved often faced problems or dilemmas that always managed to resolve to a happy ending with the 15-minute stories. With attention distracted from the noxious stimuli, though it may not completely overcome the discomfort, the individual is re-empowered to make a choice about what is the best next action. The strong value that each individual is the authority on his or her own experience was inviolable.

The power of a hug, or the presence of a calm, trusted family member significantly reduces the fear; though anyone who has worked in a hospital knows that some family members bring calm while others can amplify the fearful sensations. As a mother, I kept a private stash of fascinating games and toys for my children and would bring them forth when difficult situations presented. For an individual who seeks distraction, it can be useful to encourage pre-selection of certain books, stories, or electronic games on which to place attention.

One of the toys my son Ethan responded well to was a little stuffed bear named "Milton." Ethan knew that Milton was his own middle name, and he also knew he was named for his grandfather. Milton was a remarkable bear in that his fur unzipped, revealing pajamas underneath. I was able to capture Ethan's imagination to create the possibility that Milton's pain receptors were all on the fur, and that once he took the fur off, he was very comfortable. After we reviewed that magical capability that Milton had, Ethan laughingly engaged in gestures that mimicked him "unzipping" his own skin and removing it. That intervention helped young Ethan through a series of ear infections and stubbed toes.

The creative suggestion I offered my own son was one of a multitude of transformative or dissociative techniques that can be useful. Dad wrote about numerous cases in which dissociation was the primary tool to separate the individual from the suffering.

Can you deliberately shrink the field of conscious awareness so that it excludes the pain of an injured foot? One way anesthesia can be developed in a case with burned feet is to ask patients to forget their feet and then lose their sense of body continuity. I have inflicted painful stimuli upon a foot after such a thought without the subjects reporting stress, because they had forgotten their feet. They were naive subjects and they didn't know that I was going to pinch their feet or to inflict pain or distress on them. But they had forgotten their feet. What does that actually mean? What is amnesia? What is dissociation?

My daughter had said that under no circumstances would she ever permit anesthesia. I know my daughter's interest in hypnosis and her interest in psychology, but she was only a grade-school child at the time. I had promised her that I would not offer her any suggestion regarding anesthesia. Once in a medical setting where I was demonstrating hypnosis, I asked my daughter to see herself sitting 'over there' on the other side of the room. She was very interested in hallucinating herself 'over there.' Then I asked her to *'feel herself on the other side of the room, really to feel herself sitting there, to experience herself sitting over there.'* Then one of the doctors, over to one side came up and pinched her very thoroughly, tested her for pain. He was very certain that my daughter, experiencing herself 'over there' did not show any pain reactions. The dissociation, the hallucination of herself 'over there' was quite complete. How could she be pinched 'over here' when she was 'over there'?" (Rossi et al., 2010b, pps. 312-313)

Responses are individual; they are quite different in an individual who wants to watch, listen, notice, and explore their sensations than they are in an individual who wants to "not notice" and keep their attention drawn to areas that are more agreeable. Though the techniques may be different, pain is a strong motivator to re-align ones perceptions in a way that facilitates enjoyment of life. Dad's contagious interest in exploration and discovering new possibilities was so pronounced that it was hard to resist his invitations to try out something new. Erickson household values included admiration for hard work and discovery. Another value was making contributions to society at large, and thus, as we learned from him, there was general recognition that we would bring discoveries to others who needed them. I learned from my father to look calmly at an injury and to let curiosity guide the direction of possible interventions. I ask myself, "I wonder if it might be possible to change feeling of hurt into some other feeling?" If I am working with a patient, I verbalize this question and let their response guide the conversation further.

Erickson masterfully encouraged his children to look forward to accidents and minor medical procedures as opportunities to explore our own hypnotic capacity. Our growing skill sets prepared us to deal with significant pain should it ever enter our lives. Each opportunity to practice was celebrated; the opportunities included trips to the dentist or times when one of us stepped on a nail or brushed up against a cactus. On occasions when we worked so hard that our muscles ached, we were reminded to notice those sensations and capitalize on learning from them. Coached by our father, each of my siblings and I learned to view these occasions as wonderful opportunities—they provided a forum to examine just how far our own personal skill sets had developed to explore new hypnotic techniques for pain management. We were blessed with a ready cohort of others who appreciated the exploratory process of learning in hypnosis.

Our self-discovery as a group of siblings gave us a chance to learn at an early age that each of us responds differently to suggestions. Robert generally chose a path of distraction into a story, sometimes a book, or music. Kristi liked to get things over with quickly and was willing to accept symbolic resolution and move beyond the discomfort to invest her time and energy in ways of her own choosing. For myself, I enjoyed the intense engagement of noticing the transformation of discomfort into something different. My father worked with me closely to explore a multitude of ways to dissociate from painful stimuli. Part of my learning involved a concurrent rapt examination of steps of the process. Intervention in the interpretation of pain offers a plethora of possibilities. Individuals like myself, who are bent towards curiosity and exploration, may respond well to imaginary transformation of the stimuli into other sensations. Some individuals are immediately ready to explore the possibility of imagining that sensations have colors, sounds, come with a clear margin, or can be quantified numerically. Keeping open to possibilities expands the opportunity to engage in a playfully serious self-examination of just how potent flexibility can be. Children are particularly open to these possibilities, as if they have not yet learned the limits of what is considered to be reasonable. But playfulness need not be childish; I do not hesitate to consider the receptiveness of adults to explore magical transformation.

I recall when I got my ears pierced, at age 12. My parental permission came with a promise that I instruct the physician to not use any local anesthesia. This agreement suited me, as I had already envisioned a painless separation of my skin cells opening to allow the gold post to pass through my earlobes. I remember Dad speaking to me about minimizing bleeding or swelling and also his questioning whether I was *really ready to choose such a procedure.* I felt a sense of kinship with the local Native Americans and Mexicans who traditionally performed piercings on infants who had no recollection of the procedure. I had already spoken with my mother, who had piercing done as an adult, and she used what I consider a distraction technique; but I myself wanted to turn my attention towards the sensation and actually feel the movement of the cells as they stepped aside. I walked alone to the physician's office; part of my parent's style of encouraging independence and self-responsibility. By the time I experienced the procedure, I was captivated by noting the sensation of the cells parting. When it was over, I was surprised by the sound of the needle and thrilled with my own success.

One additional technique that can significantly enhance success is time distortion and pseudo-orientation in time. When Erickson moved the conversation with Robert forward, exploring the interactions between Robert and his cut lip, Robert began participating actively in the resolution of the injury. Likewise, his encouragement that we look forward to dental visits as an opportunity to see ourselves successful is another way of future projection that gives us practice in moving past the moment into a sensation of healing.

> Pain is a complex, a construct, composed of past remembered pain, of present pain experience, and of anticipated pain of the future. Thus, immediate pain is augmented by past pain and of the future. The immediate stimuli are only a central third of the entire experience. Nothing so much intensifies pain as the fear

that it will be present on the morrow. It is likewise increased by the realization that the same or similar pain was experienced in the past, and this and the immediate pain render the future even more threatening. Conversely the realization that the present pain is a single event which will come definitely to a pleasant ending serves greatly to diminish pain. Because pain is a complex, a construct, it is more readily vulnerable to hypnosis as a modality of dealing successfully with it than it would be if it were simply an experience of the present." (Rossi et al., 2010c, p. 96)

A beautiful resolution to a case I worked on was with a gentleman, Walter, who had excruciatingly painful phantom limb pain secondary to amputation for a terminal malignancy. Walter was a frequent visitor to the Emergency Room (ER) and the team responded quickly with medications that had previously served to alleviate his discomfort. On one occasion, his pain was untouched by the narcotics and his cries of distress continued to amplify. It was only after the personnel had exhausted their options and were frustrated with the disruption that his ongoing screams created in the ER that they called me in from another department to see whether I could help him with hypnosis.

My immediate response was to rush to the patient's side; I held onto his hand. My calm presence allowed him to consider the possibility that I might be able to help him. My previous contact with the patient facilitated his trust that I would be able to direct his energy in ways that he valued—I already knew that he really hoped to spend his final days with a beloved niece and to be able to teach her some of what he had learned in life. The niece was there, crying in a chair distant from the gurney on which he lay. I leaned over and whispered in his ear, "Remember a time before your leg was painful."

With his attention captured, I encouraged him to review with me what it felt like to be pain free, to walk on two legs. The pseudo-orientation in time to an experience of comfort was all that was needed to get him through the moment. I will never forget the calm that washed over his face. That transformational moment opened the door for capturing more days in which quality of life prevailed. Months later, after Walter had passed away, the niece sought me out to report that the remainder of his life had been peaceful.

Learning from the patients themselves is the most valuable kind of learning. Erickson's own experiences with pain following polio and the lifelong ramifications of ongoing neurological pain and muscle wasting gave him first-hand knowledge. He transformed his own experiences into creative opportunities to intervene in the ways that one responds to pain. My own professional path brought me in contact with large numbers of individuals who suffered from physical injuries or illnesses. In my upbringing, I witnessed many patients whom Dad treated for pain. With some of them he would talk about their work, with some he would talk about radio shows, what they enjoyed, or what their future hopes would be. Other times, he offered long, drawn-out stories that seemed unrelated to the injury or discomfort at hand. No case or situation was identical to his previous work—rather each case focused on individual interests, needs, and strengths.

While it is a disservice to ignore or disregard a body sensation without attending to the important signal that has been transmitted, effective care involves a balance of noticing, accepting, attending, and then putting the sensations in the larger context of a comfortable and healthy lifestyle.

Techniques, whether intended for chronic or acute pain, are not so distinct as individual situations are. Erickson brings us once again to the potency of hypnosis to serve others in pain.

> Hypnosis, by permitting the individual to call upon and utilize singly or collectively the great multitude of bodily learnings accumulated in a fragmentary fashion over the years, offers endless opportunity... to single out and examine individual manifestations. In this way hypnosis offers a means of reaching an eventual understanding of the processes entering into the development, of various behavioral phenomena. (Rossi et al., 2010b, p. 343)

Over time, we have seen the many ways that Erickson's studies have had a positive impact on medical care as well as on the quality of life of those with whom he worked. It is our time, and our turn, to reach out and share what we learn as we continue this important work.

References

Rossi, E., Erickson-Klein, R., & Rossi, K. (Eds). (2008a). *The collected works of Milton H. Erickson (Vol. 1): The nature of therapeutic hypnosis.* Phoenix, AZ: The Erickson Foundation Press.

Rossi, E., Erickson-Klein, R., & Rossi, K. (Eds). (2008b). *The collected works of Milton H. Erickson (Vol. 2): Basis hypnotic induction and suggestion.* Phoenix, AZ: The Erickson Foundation Press.

Rossi, E., Erickson-Klein, R., & Rossi, K. (Eds). (2008c). *The collected works of Milton H. Erickson (Vol. 3): Opening the mind: Innovative psychotherapy.* Phoenix, AZ: The Erickson Foundation Press.

Rossi, E., Erickson-Klein, R., & Rossi, K. (Eds). (2008d). *The collected works of Milton H. Erickson (Vol. 4): Advanced approaches to therapeutic hypnosis.* Phoenix, AZ: The Erickson Foundation Press.

Rossi, E., Erickson-Klein, R., & Rossi, K. (Eds). (2010a). *The collected works of Milton H. Erickson (Vol. 5): Classical hypnotic phenomena, Part 1: Psychodynamics.* Phoenix, AZ: The Erickson Foundation Press.

Rossi, E., Erickson-Klein, R., & Rossi, K. (Eds). (2010b). *The collected works of Milton H. Erickson (Vol. 6): Classical hypnotic phenomena, Part 2: Memory and hallucinations.* Phoenix, AZ: The Erickson Foundation Press.

Rossi, E., Erickson-Klein, R., & Rossi, K. (Eds). (2010c). *The collected works of Milton H. Erickson (Vol. 7): Mind body healing and rehabilitation.* Phoenix, AZ: The Erickson Foundation Press.

Rossi, E., Erickson-Klein, R., & Rossi, K. (Eds). (2010d). *The collected works of Milton H. Erickson (Vol. 8): General and historical surveys of hypnosis.* Phoenix, AZ: The Erickson Foundation Press.

Rossi, E., Erickson-Klein, R., & Rossi, K. (Eds). (2009). *The collected works of Milton H. Erickson (Vol. 9): The February man.* Phoenix, AZ: The Erickson Foundation Press.

Rossi, E., Erickson-Klein, R., & Rossi, K. (Eds). (2010e). *The collected works of Milton H. Erickson (Vol. 10): Hypnotic realities.* Phoenix, AZ: The Erickson Foundation Press.

Rossi, E., Erickson-Klein, R., & Rossi, K. (Eds). (2014a). *The collected works of Milton H. Erickson (Vol. 11): Hypnotherapy: An exploratory casebook.* Phoenix, AZ: The Erickson Foundation Press.

Rossi, E., Erickson-Klein, R., & Rossi, K. (Eds). (2014b). *The collected works of Milton H. Erickson (Vol. 12): Experiencing hypnosis: Therapeutic approaches to altered states.* Phoenix, AZ: The Erickson Foundation Press.

Rossi, E., Erickson-Klein, R., & Rossi, K. (Eds). (2014c). *The collected works of Milton H. Erickson (Vol. 13): Healing in hypnosis: Seminars, workshops and lectures, Part 1.* Phoenix, AZ: The Erickson Foundation Press.

Rossi, E., Erickson-Klein, R., & Rossi, K. (Eds). (2014d). *The collected works of Milton H. Erickson (Vol. 14): Life reframing in hypnosis: Seminars, workshops and lectures, Part 2.* Phoenix, AZ: The Erickson Foundation Press.

Rossi, E., Erickson-Klein, R., & Rossi, K. (Eds). (2015a). *The collected works of Milton H. Erickson (Vol. 15): Mind body communication in hypnosis: Seminars, workshops and lectures, Part 3.* Phoenix, AZ: The Erickson Foundation Press.

Rossi, E., Erickson-Klein, R., & Rossi, K. (Eds). (2015b). *The collected works of Milton H. Erickson (Vol. 16): Creative choice in hypnosis: Seminars, workshops and lectures, Part 4.* Phoenix, AZ: The Erickson Foundation Press.

CHAPTER 10

Hypnotic Management of Surgery-Related Pain

Audrey Vanhaudenhuyse and
Marie-Elisabeth Faymonville

Marie-Elisabeth Faymonville is a physician specializing in anesthesia and intensive care medicine. In 1992, she developed a new method of anesthesia, named hypnosedation. Since 1994, she has been teaching hypnosis and hypnotic techniques at the University of Liège, Wallonia, Belgium. Her research originally focused on the investigation of the neuroanatomical mechanisms of various states of consciousness, including hypnosis. As a professor, she heads the Algology and Palliative Care Department of the University Hospital of Liège. Her clinical approach, using hypnosis in surgery, chronic pain, oncology, and palliative care has enabled her to promote hypnosis as a tool in modern medicine.

Audrey Vanhaudenhuyse, PhD, is a neuropsychologist. She works in the Algology and Palliative Care Department of the University Hospital of Liège and heads the Sensation and Perception GIGA Research Group of the University of Liège. Her research program studies modified states of consciousness, including hypnosis, in patients with chronic pain, cancer, and altered states of consciousness (coma, unresponsive wakefulness syndrome/

vegetative state, minimally conscious state). Her work includes neurophysiological studies which seek to better understand the brain mechanisms that underlie the beneficial effects of hypnosis and other states of consciousness.

* * *

Surgery is a major cause of acute pain. In 1846, the first anesthetic provided pain-free surgery. One hundred and seventy-two years later, patients should not have to endure unrelieved pain in hospital; the relief of such pain is of the utmost importance to anyone treating patients who are undergoing surgery.

Efficient pain management is fundamental to ensure quality of care, since appropriate pain relief leads to shortened hospital stays, reduced hospital costs, and increased patient satisfaction (Garimella & Cellini, 2013). Although improvements in pharmacological interventions have greatly improved surgical recovery, these methods are still not perfect and are often associated with negative side effects such as post-operative nausea and vomiting, as well as cognitive disorders. These adverse events, related to the use of analgesic medications, can be associated with impaired performance of activities of daily living (Moller et al., 1998), premature withdrawal from the labor market (Steinmetz et al., 2009), and deterioration of quality of life (Newman et al., 2001). There are, therefore, obvious social and financial reasons for patients to be able to experience maximum comfort with minimal adverse events.

Hypnosis in the Surgical Theatre

Starting over 25 years ago, in 1992, we began using hypnosis as an adjunct to mild conscious sedation (also known as hypnosedation) when performing surgery with local anesthesia. This technique was first used in the Plastic Surgery Department of the University Hospital of Liège (Belgium) as surgeons routinely used local anesthesia and patients were interested in avoiding general anesthesia (Faymonville et al., 1995). Due to an overwhelmingly positive experience, hypnosedation has been used, since 1994, for various surgical and assessment procedures, including thyroid surgery, vascular and renal procedures, breast and prostate biopsy, mammary adenomectomies, colectomy, implant sterilization placement, tooth extraction, skin tumor removal, labor and childbirth, glioma surgery, and burn dressing change (for a review, see Vanhaudenhuyse et al., 2014).

Use of hypnosedation is associated with improved peri- and post-operative comfort, as well as with better conditions during the performance of surgery, when compared with general anesthesia (Meurisse et al., 1999). Studies have also shown that hypnosedation is associated with reductions in anxiety, emotional distress, pain, and nausea, as well as diminished intraoperative requirements for anxiolytic and analgesic drugs (Defechereux et al., 2000; Faymonville et al., 1999). Some studies have also shown a faster post-operative recovery (Tefikow et al., 2013), with, for example, significant decreases in back-to-work times (Defechereux et al., 1999, 2000).

The procedure is carried out as follows. In the Surgery Department of the University Hospital of Liège, surgeons inform patients about the possibility of performing the elected surgery with hypnosedation, as an alternative to general anesthesia. Deafness, dementia, severe psychiatric disorders, and allergies to local anesthetics are exclusion criteria. Informed consent is the first requirement for inclusion.

The surgical decision to operate with hypnosedation and local anesthesia depends on the surgeon's own appreciation of its feasibility with the particular case in question, as well as the usual routines associated with the relevant type of surgery. Indeed, hypnosedation modifies the working conditions: the patient is conscious during the entire procedure, and the team must communicate well and work closely together throughout the procedure.

With hypnosedation, the pre-operative anesthetic interview includes a detailed medical and surgical history, drug consumption history, and clinical examination. After the initial interview, the anesthesiologist asks the patient about his or her motivation for agreeing to have hypnosedation and then provides a thorough description of the various stages of the planned anesthetic and surgical procedures, as well as information about conscious intravenous sedation. Furthermore, this consultation aims to describe the hypnotic state and creates an atmosphere in which the patient feels free to ask any questions.

No "dry run" is proposed or performed. The anesthesiologist emphasizes that motivation, confidence, and collaboration with the medical team are essential for success. The patient knows that they will place themselves in the hypnotic state and that they will be distracted from surgery while remaining conscious.

On the day of surgery, in the operating room, monitoring for vital signs is initiated and an intravenous line is installed. A hypnotic state is then induced using eye fixation, muscle relaxation, and permissive and indirect suggestions. The safe-place metaphor (presented below as a typical script) is used by the anesthesiologist.

However, the specific suggestions during the course of the induction vary depending upon the anesthesiologist's observations of a patient's behaviors and needs. When the patient is thought to be at an adequate level of trance (after three to ten minutes, when slow eye movements are observed), the psychological approach is supplemented by intravenous administration of small amounts of remifentanil. This helps to maintain the patient in a conscious state, increases analgesia, and provides comfortable and quiet surgical conditions.

Local anesthesia provided by the surgeon is then performed. Throughout surgery, the anesthesiologist speaks with the patient in a monotonous voice, using metaphors.

At the end of the procedure, the anesthesiologist, using his or her normal voice, invites the patient to re-establish contact with the outside world. This serves to restore a normal state of consciousness in just a few seconds. The patient is then transferred to the ward where oral intake (of water, or if desired by the patient, food) is immediately allowed and oral analgesics are administered when or if the patient requests them.

The "Safe-Place" Metaphor

When the patient arrives at the operating room, I greet him or her and then ask, "Are you ready to work with me?" Then, as the patient is moved to the operating table, and while we prepare and place the vital signs monitoring equipment, I suggest, "While we put in place everything that is useful for your safety, I suggest that you think about something nice that you want to experience during the surgery." Thus, while I place the catheter for the intravenous drip, the patient can silently explore his or her "good moments" video library.

I ask the patient to, "Give me the information that you think would be useful for me to be able to accompany you adequately during surgery." The nurse helps me to ensure that the patient is comfortably prepared for the surgery. I then begin the hypnotic induction.

Anesthesiologist: I invite you now to take a moment to find a comfortable position, with your head comfortably supported, so that you can look at something here in the room for a period of time; some object in the room or a specific point on the wall. Take the time to pay attention to the finest details of this object... noticing the changes that suddenly appear as you pay close attention to the object. Observe its colors, its shape, its texture... and discover that changes appear. Perhaps at some point the outlines begin to blur, or maybe the shadows mix in with the colors, to give them a new intensity.

Perhaps you are noticing the colors changing with the light around this object or point. Perhaps the way that you are looking at the object or point can even make the shadows change... sometimes the object or point might disappear and reappear... or change in some other way.

You might start to feel changes in the eyes. You may notice a minor tickling in the eyes... or maybe a tension in the eye muscles, in the face muscles. You can soothe these sensations by slowly relaxing the face muscles... all of them, including those around the eyes. Letting the eyes slowly close... to relax your sight and your eyes.

You can now see, behind your closed eyelids, different colors... different shapes... and different shadows. Follow them closely... and you realize that here too, changes appear as you focus on these colors, shapes, and shadows. ... These

changes continue and you realize that they bring to you a certain peace of mind. ... This inner peace reminds you, perhaps, of a special place buried deep inside your memory. ... Your safe place.

> [I then signal to the nurse that she or he can sterilize the surgical field, and I say to the patient:]

And while we are washing, you maybe discover in your place, a place, a moment, or a freshness that helps you increase your comfort. My voice accompanies you... and you can transform my words into those you need to hear; words that you find most useful and comforting.

This memory, this place, slowly comes back to you and you start to see elements of it. ... Slowly, the details of this wonderful place... inside your memory... come back to you, and settle into your current reality.

You find yourself slowly transported back into your safe place. As you slowly approach your peaceful place, you may hear certain sounds that invite you, deeper and deeper, back into this place. Listen closely to these sounds, maybe they're the sounds of nature... or maybe even the sound of silence.

Let these sounds guide you deeper into your experience. It now seems that everything comes back to you, even the air that you are breathing reminds you of that particular place... deep inside your memory.

And while we place some tissues [briefly describing any preparatory procedures that are happening at this juncture] here, you can discover even more details of your place. Perhaps you notice a fragrance; it smells pure... and fresh. You notice the sights... the sounds, and the smells... everything that you notice brings you a feeling of peace... the peacefulness of this place.

Taking the time you need to observe the details of this beautiful place... being aware of the wonderful atmosphere, as we adjust the light of the scialytic lamp...

[Note: A scialytic lamp is the lamp that illuminates the surgical field.]

Perhaps you notice how the light changes colors... with the coming and going of seasons, and, as a result, start to appreciate the abundance of certain beautiful and absorbing colors in this particular place.

You are able see colors everywhere... how they blend and how they change. When you look at what is around you in detail, it invites you to take time for yourself... the time you need. ... And as you do this, you are allowing yourself to rediscover the sensations that are particularly familiar to you in this specific place; perhaps it's the temperature that surrounds you, or a particularly comfortable sensation that you feel, like when a ray of sunlight comes to smoothly warm your skin...

And while numbing the site for your comfort...

[The surgeon injects local anesthesia into the surgical field.]

you discover different elements of the nature that surrounds you. You can enjoy the fresh air you are breathing, just like you can enjoy a cool breeze passing by, cooling you off in the warmth of the sun, and other elements of nature that you enjoy in your place... letting yourself feel, live, and appreciate the little elements that are important to you in this special place.

Perhaps this element is water; fresh water that you hear flowing, not very far away, making its way into the depths of nature. These important elements might also be the colors, their abundance, and the masterpiece that they create by blending together in their unique way. Or perhaps the single most important element is the sound you hear; perhaps even the beautiful sound of silence. Continuing to allow your beautiful, unique, and safe place deep inside your memory to sing to you... the lullaby of nature.

Letting yourself experience the little things you enjoy about this place. Perhaps you find that what you are looking at is part of many other places... you can appreciate the color of a stone... the contact with and sensation of this stone. ... It may be pleasant to touch the bark of a tree, to feel in this contact a link, a link with the roots of this tree and the earth around it. Perhaps contact with other elements that are found in nature can be deeply satisfying, like the smoothness of water or the freshness and comfort of the morning grass on which you walk barefoot.

These variations of color in nature, with the light changing the colors as the day goes by, as the seasons go by. These changes allow you to find in your place, in your safe place, everything you need to feel perfectly comfortable, to enjoy the softness of the sensations that this place brings to you, how safe you feel inside it, letting yourself fully appreciate all the amazing feelings that your place brings to you.

Letting yourself slowly discover, perhaps, your favorite season, the beautiful light that it brings, and how it brings everything to life, brings the colors out and draws everything around you in the most beautiful colors which bring to you the best feelings you know.

[If the patient grimaces as a way to communicate local discomfort, I report this to the surgeon by using the word "uncomfort." The surgeon then may inject a local anesthetic or loosen the tissue traction.]

Sometimes, being able to move, feeling your body in contact with the earth, the consistency of the earth on which your feet walk... at other moments it may be more the atmosphere that you are breathing... whatever stands out... of all that you hear and feel... all that you experience. Letting yourself enjoy this wonderful moment like a gift, a wonderful gift from life itself...

And this gift gives you the ability to recharge from the endless energy of nature, like you could enjoy feeling refreshed with cool water, or enjoy drinking something delicious, enjoying the taste and scent of it. You stay in this place, enjoying the details of everything that surrounds you, taking the time you need to discover what is important for you to discover. And realizing that whenever it would be important for you to find this feeling again, your safe place is always available... and can provide for you what you seek.

This harmony, this peace of mind, and this balance that you are feeling right now, it is available anytime and anywhere, in your safe place. Your safe place provides you with an endlessly powerful tool to feel well within yourself, within your environment, and with the people around you. As of right now, you are enriched, having taken a beautiful trip to your favorite place, a moment of total inner peace; with the knowledge that this experience is available to you whenever it would be useful to you. Use this tool, this ability to go to your safe place, as often as you need... to feel more in harmony with yourself and with your surroundings.

[At the end of the surgical procedure, using my normal voice, I invite the patient to reestablish contact with the operating theater.]

Now, slowly, you can decide to get back in touch with feeling the support with which you started this exercise... you can begin to move your body again... to regain contact with reality... with the here and now.

And when you are fully in touch with your body, when you are fully back into this reality, at that moment, you know that when you open your eyes, the exercise is over... you are feeling fresh and ready, able to do everything that you need to do... at the moment that you decide to do it.

Final Comments

Intra-operative conversion from hypnosedation to general anesthesia has only occurred in 18 out of about 9500 (0.2%) patients that have been treated to date. These conversions were due to a variety of reasons, including positional discomfort (e.g., neck hyperextension), lack of sufficient pain relief, more complicated surgical procedures, or anxiety upon the induction of hypnosis. There have been no deaths and no other specific morbidity related to the use of this technique.

On the other hand, hypnosedation has resulted in high patient satisfaction and better recovery. It can be used in most motivated patients and reduces the socio-economic impact of hospitalization. This technique can be performed safely, efficiently, and cost-effectively. We therefore propose this technique as a valuable alternative to standard anesthetic protocols for certain surgical procedures. The major benefit of this technique is to maximize patient comfort during surgery, while also avoiding pharmacological unconsciousness. The active participation of the patient in optimizing their own recovery appears to be a significant factor in the consistent patient satisfaction we have observed.

However, this technique imposes a change in the function and focus of the surgical team. As the patient remains conscious throughout surgery, previously inconsequential details such as tissue manipulation, noise levels, and conversation among the surgical team must be considered. The surgical team and the anesthesiologist are obliged to monitor the surgical procedure and to constantly take into account the patient's physical and psychological needs. These requirements may represent a considerable change in the working habits of a surgical team.

There is no longer any doubt regarding the neurophysiological basis for the hypnotic state and its acceptance in the scientific community. Therefore, any logistical problems should be addressed in the interests of the patient's comfort and health. The success of this technique depends on the surgeon's technical skills and ability to concentrate, the commitment of the entire surgical team, and a willingness of the team to change established habits in order to benefit the patient.

References

Defechereux, T., Degauque, C., Fumal, I., Faymonville, M. E., Joris, J., Hamoir, E., & Meurisse, M. (2000). L'hypnosédation, un nouveau mode d'anesthésie pour la chirurgie endocrinienne cervicale. Étude prospective randomisée [Hypnosedation, a new method of anesthesia for cervical endocrine surgery. Prospective randomized study]. *Annales De Chirurgie, 125*, 539-546.

Defechereux, T., Meurisse, M., Hamoir, E., Gollogly, L., Joris, J., & Faymonville, M. E. (1999). Hypnoanesthesia for endocrine cervical surgery: A statement of practice. *Journal of Alternative and Complementary Medicine, 5*, 509-520.

Faymonville, M. E., Fissette, J., Mambourg, P. H., Roediger, L., Joris, J., & Lamy, M. (1995). Hypnosis as adjunct therapy in conscious sedation for plastic surgery. *Regional Anesthesia, 20*, 145-151.

Faymonville, M. E., Meurisse, M., & Fissette, J. (1999). Hypnosedation: A valuable alternative to traditional anesthetic techniques. *Acta Chirurgica Belgica, 99*, 141-146.

Garimella, V., & Cellini, C. (2013). Postoperative pain control. *Clinics in Colon and Rectal Surgery, 26*, 191-196.

Meurisse, M., Defechereux, T., Hamoir, E., Maweja, S., Marchettini, P., Gollogly, L., ... Faymonville, M. E. (1999). Hypnosis with conscious sedation instead of general anesthesia? Applications in cervical endocrine surgery. *Acta Chirurgica Belgica, 99*, 151-158.

Moller, J. T., Cluitmans, P., Rasmussen, L. S., Houx, P., Rasmussen, H., Canet, J., ... Gravenstein, J. S. (1998). Long-term postoperative cognitive dysfunction in the elderly ISPOCD1 study. ISPOCD investigators. International Study of Post-Operative Cognitive Dysfunction. *Lancet, 351*, 857-861.

Newman, M. F., Grocott, H. P., Mathew, J. P., White, W. D., Landolfo, K., Reves, J. G., ... Blumenthal, J. A. (2001). Report of the substudy assessing the impact of neurocognitive function on quality of life 5 years after cardiac surgery. *Stroke, 32*, 2874-2881.

Steinmetz, J., Christensen, K. B., Lund, T., Lohse, N., Rasmussen, L. S., & ISPOCD Group. (2009). Long-term consequences of postoperative cognitive dysfunction. *Anesthesiology, 110,* 548-555.

Tefikow, S., Barth, J., Maichrowitz, S., Beelmann, A., Strauss, B., & Rosendahl, J. (2013). Efficacy of hypnosis in adults undergoing surgery or medical procedures: A meta-analysis of randomized controlled trials. *Clinical Psychology Review, 33,* 623-636.

Vanhaudenhuyse, A., Laureys, S., & Faymonville, M. E. (2014). Neurophysiology of hypnosis. *Neurophysiologie Clinique/Clinical Neurophysiology, 44,* 343-353.

CHAPTER 11

Hypnosis for Dental Procedures

Michael Alan Gow

Mike Gow is a general dental practitioner working in private practice at The Berkeley Clinic in Glasgow, UK. He graduated from Glasgow University in 1999. His interest in hypnosis was sparked while he was still a dental student, and he completed his basic hypnosis training in 2001. In 2005, he graduated with a master's degree in Hypnosis Applied to Dentistry from the University of London, having achieved a Distinction at the Diploma level. He has a postgraduate certificate in the Management of Dental Anxiety from the University of Edinburgh. Mike is a past president of The British Society of Medical & Dental Hypnosis (Scotland) and is a founding member of The International Society of Dental Anxiety Management. Mike holds the European Certificate of Hypnosis and has published dozens of papers and cases on the topic of hypnosis. He regularly attends and presents at hypnosis workshops and conferences throughout the world.

Mike has appeared on television several times to demonstrate the use of hypnosis in place of local anesthetics for controlling pain during invasive dental procedures, including: a dental filling (BBC's Exposed- Persuaders), removal of a wisdom tooth (BBC's Horizon) sinus lift and implant placement (More4's Hypnosurgery Live), and immediate placement implants (BBC's Alternative

Therapies). He has also appeared on radio documentaries for the BBC's World Service.

* * *

Pain is a wonderful thing. Without pain, very few species of animals, including Homo sapiens, could survive. Pain protects us from burning ourselves with fire, plunging our hands into boiling or freezing water, cutting ourselves with knives, and a variety of other potentially traumatic or life-threatening injuries and situations. It helps us protect previously injured body parts from further injury, assists healing, and warns us of disease.

A dental abscess or acute pulpitis can result in extremely unpleasant experiences; however, the pain associated with these conditions signals to us that there is a dental problem that needs attention. When pain has such signal value, it really is one of the most useful results of evolution.

The trouble is, pain is far more complex than just an objective, reactive, or warning signal that keeps us safe. Pain experiences vary between individuals; what may be tolerable for one person may be intolerable for another. The subjective experience is affected by biological variation, memory, anticipation, expectations, anxiety, and a variety of other factors. These factors evolve as they help give our sensory experience context—allowing the brain to distinguish sensations that indicate danger from those that that are just... sensations. This further protects us from risk of injury or death.

Despite its necessity for our survival, pain remains an unpleasant experience. Indeed, the word *pain* has its roots in the same words inferring punishment such as penalty, penance, and penitentiary. A dental bur burrowing into a tooth, or forceps applied with sufficient force to avulse a tooth from its socket, will create the experience of pain in the absence of an anesthetic. The brain, understandably, interprets these as trauma and therefore signals danger.

In the last few hundred years however, such traumatic dental and medical interventions, whose purpose is to heal and prolong quality of life, have advanced dramatically. With the advent of pharmacological analgesics and anesthetics we entered a new era. Without this science, many of the procedures that are now considered routine (such as most of dentistry) would simply not have been possible in the relatively recent past.

Early in 2001, having only recently completed the basic training in hypnosis, I was presented with an interesting case. An elderly lady had severe facial pain on the right side. All dental investigations ruled out a dental cause and a referral was made to the local hospital. Eventually, a consultant report returned concluding that her pain was likely of psychogenic origin.

I explained to the patient that this meant that they believed that while the experience of her pain was as real as if there was a physical cause, no physical cause was evident. She asked if there was anything I could do. I told her that I had recently trained in hypnosis and that this was an effective approach for some people in at least reducing or managing their experience of pain. Bearing in mind that I was 24 years old at the time, she was understandably dubious and declined. (As I recall, her exact words were, "Hypnosis? No chance son!").

Some three months later her husband returned, explaining that her pain was worsening. She rarely left her house and struggled to sleep, with the pain often reducing her to tears. He explained that she had seen consultants and pain specialists and had explored a variety of complementary and alternative approaches, but that nothing had helped. He then said that his wife had asked him to enquire about the hypnosis I had mentioned.

In hearing the list of failed approaches, I felt my heart sink. I was concerned about over-promising and under-delivering. Despite this, and wanting to help, I advised that she make an appointment for us to talk about the possibilities of hypnosis. She duly arrived for her appointment a couple of weeks later but was in tears as she entered my consultation room. She explained that the pain was particularly bad that day and that she had nearly cancelled the appointment. I decided to put my plan of a lengthy assessment and discussion about hypnosis to the side. After a brief assessment to ensure that there were no contraindications to hypnosis, and with her consent, I undertook a 30-minute hypnosis session.

After induction, I taught her to enter her "special place," which she chose to be a garden in the summer. After enjoying this place and relaxing for a while, I introduced her to the "comfort dial" (see specific script later in this chapter). With this technique, while hypnotized, the patient is to construct an image of a dial that reports and controls their level of comfort. There are numbers around the dial up to 10, with 0 being totally comfortable, and 10 being the most discomfort (or pain) imaginable. The imagined dial is to be something controllable, such as a volume control on a stereo, the dial on a safe, the speedometer on a car, or a shower valve. At the start of the technique, the patient is to report the number currently displayed. In this case, the patient reported an 8 out of 10.

Following the advice that I had picked up from reading the work of Kay Thompson (cf. Kane & Olness, 2004;

Thompson, 1963, 1977), I first acknowledged this by saying, "Wow, that must really hurt." This first statement is important as it ensures that the patient knows that you understand the severity of their experience and have empathy.

I then asked, "Would you like to learn how you can make it better?" This question implies that "making it better" is a possibility and that the control to do so belongs to the patient themselves, once learned. Use of the word *better* is important as well. *Better* can be interpreted as complete resolution (e.g., "I was ill, but now I'm better now"), but can also imply improvement without complete resolution (e.g., "I am still ill, but I am better than I was").

I then asked her to focus on the number 8, and with her consent for a very short spell only, to see if she could turn this number up to an 8½ or a 9. As she did this, her increased discomfort was visible by her facial expression. She was then invited to turn the number back down again so that it was "only an 8." The word *only* is important here as it suggests that the 8 is now a more manageable, smaller number in comparison.

After she increased and decreased her pain intensity in this way several times, she was invited to then turn the number down to a 7. She was able to do this quite easily. I then asked her which number would mean that she could get on with her day unimpeded, and I invited her to lower her dial to this number or lower. After a few minutes, she reported that it was now at a number 3 and she was happy. After the session, I taught her self-hypnosis and we booked another appointment. Over the years, I have also adapted the comfort dial for use in controlling acute pain during dental procedures.

Prior to her next appointment, I read up on several pain control techniques and spoke to various mentors. I planned a lengthy session that would investigate possible causes and that would offer her a variety of pain control techniques. The day arrived and I sat with all my notes ready as she entered my room. The first thing she said to me as she came in however was, "I'm really sorry, you're going to be really annoyed with me." I was concerned by this and asked her why she thought that I would be annoyed. She explained that she thought the 90-minute session would be a waste of time. I asked her why she thought this, and I was genuinely taken aback when she replied, "Because after the last session, the pain started to come back so I used the self-hypnosis. I turned the dial down, and got it to 0. There was a click and the pain went away. That was two weeks ago and it hasn't been back." She felt bad for me that she was wasting the appointment but had not wanted to cancel in case it had come back!

She was like a different person that day, and the pain never returned. While I was already impressed by what I had seen and experienced following my basic hypnosis training, after this experience I felt compelled to study hypnosis to a greater level. Pain control is probably the area of hypnosis which has had the most research, the most media interest (it can certainly make for compelling television), and can create the most dramatic and sensational effects. Hypnotic analgesia has a long history and is arguably one of the earliest applications of hypnosis in dentistry (Chaves 1997).

To date, I have been involved in several cases using hypnosis alone (i.e., without anesthetics), including dental restoration surgery, dental extractions, a sinus lift, and implant placements. Some of these cases were recorded for television and radio documentaries. These cases reinforced to me the potential benefits of hypnosis for pain control in dentistry (Gow & Faqir, 2008; Gow, 2010).

As a "wet fingered" dentist, like every other dentist, I have to manage patients' expectations and experience of acute pain multiple times on a daily basis. Each case has to be managed on an individual basis and each will have a different combination of techniques and approaches. I apply the skills that I have learned from training in hypnosis in an informal way in just about every case I encounter.

"The practitioner who is competently trained in hypnosis will find that there is a diminished need for the use of hypnosis *per se*, with most of his patients (Stolzenburg, 1961)." The rationale behind this statement is that in studying rapport, language, communication, and suggestion for effective hypnosis, the practitioner finds that these skills can be enough, when combined with simple relaxation or distraction techniques, even without a formal trance to help create change in many situations. Those who have studied the work of Dr. Milton Erickson know that these are probably the most important clinical skills that you can ever learn and develop (see Chapter 9, this volume).

A Few Important Tips for Language in the Dental Environment

We know that increased anxiety can lead to an increased experience of pain. Therefore, it makes sense that any language technique to help reduce anxiety will be of benefit. If your reception staff tells patients, "I'm sorry, the dentist is running late" then the patient's confidence in you is lowered and their anxiety may become higher, potentially resulting in a lower pain tolerance. If you are indeed running behind schedule, ask your reception staff to replace the previous statement with, "The dentist knows that you are here and has asked me to let you know that s/he is having to take a little longer to help the person before you. S/he has asked me to make sure that you are aware of the short delay and to make sure you are OK for time today. Is there anything I can do or get for you to make you more comfortable in the meantime?"

In addition, it is useful to avoid using emotive words. Translating emotive words such as *drill* to *handpiece, pain* to *pressure, drilling* to *buzzing, long needle* to *block, waiting room* to *lounge* or *sitting room, extract* to *remove,* and *surgery* to *treatment room* are prime examples of changes that can easily be made in your daily language. Remember also that any translation should be age appropriate for the patient.

Note that it is important that patients are aware that they will still feel pressure, temperature, and movement. To promise that they will feel *nothing* sets up unrealistic expectations, is inaccurate, and would therefore be counterproductive. Avoid promising *no pain,* because when or if the patient feels any discomfort, their expectation of pain and anxiety will increase as their trust decreases.

The word *try* should be avoided as it implies failure (Ewin, 2009). "Try to relax" implies that the patient will fail or at least find relaxing very difficult. "Allow yourself to relax" is far more likely to result in the desired effect, while remaining permissive.

Avoid negative language when possible (Gow, 2008). If I ask you, for example, to **not** think about an elephant at any point in the next 30 seconds it may surprise you that you find you can think of little else. If I ask you to **not** think about whether it is an Indian or African elephant, you would find it difficult to avoid thinking of one or other (or both!). The task becomes harder if I also ask that you should **not** even think about a toy elephant (either pink or blue) or a wooden carving of an elephant. Do **not** wonder whether the tusks in the wooden elephant are plastic or real ivory. Do **not** think about elephants at all in any way. So, it is almost impossible not to think of elephants isn't it? With this in mind, consider now the things dentists and the dental team say every day to our patients: "Don't worry, it won't hurt." It is clear how patients who hear such language can remain anxious and focus **more** on their experience of pain. Consider a simple translation to: "Allow yourself to relax and this will be surprisingly comfortable."

Dissociation often helps when working with anxious patients, especially when emotive words are also translated. Changing the word *your* to *the* can actually have quite a noticeable dissociative effect. Rather than saying, "I'm going to extract your tooth today," say "The tooth will be removed today." Rather than saying, "**You** might experience swelling, bruising, pain, or numbness..." consider saying instead, "**Some people** might experience some swelling, bruising, discomfort, or numbness..." The information communicated in these statements is the same; however, the patient's emotive response can be very different due to how they process the information.

Linguistic techniques such as these can be utilized when considering information leaflets and when obtaining informed consent. With these techniques, you will perhaps consider how your patients can be given written and verbal information in order to make an informed decision in a way that avoids overly concerning or upsetting them, especially prior to a treatment that has the potential to be uncomfortable.

During a routine restorative dental procedure, I tend to use the following protocol:

1. Ensure good rapport with the patient and use language and communication techniques to minimize anxiety throughout the procedure.

2. Apply topical anesthetic for at least 90 seconds.

3. Administer local anesthetic comfortably and slowly, preferably with a computer-controlled system such as The Wand STA (Milestone Scientific, Livingstone, NJ). Use distraction and relaxation techniques throughout (Gow, 2006a, 2006b).

4. Allow sufficient time for any anesthetic administered to work.

5. In every case, I will test the anesthesia. In reality, what I do is touch the tooth once with the dental bur and then immediately stop and ask the patient if the experience was comfortable. As the test involves very little in the way of stimulus that would cause pain, it gives the patient a reduced expectation of pain from further exposure to the treatment and lowers anxiety. In the event of a patient reporting pain, I would consider further anesthetic but also assess and address their level of anxiety and expectation.

6. As the treatment begins, word substitution to replace emotive and negative words as outlined previously can be effective (e.g., "Be aware that there will be a lot of pressure as the tooth is removed, it can be quite an unusual and interesting feeling.")

I am continually striving to learn new strategies and techniques to help make the experience of dental treatment more comfortable for my patients. It is my hope that this chapter will add to your own armamentarium. Over the years, I have learned many great techniques and gained valuable ideas from hypnosis workshops, lectures, books, and publications that were not in fact specifically about dentistry. If you are a dentist and you have skipped straight to this chapter, make sure you read the rest of this book!

Rapid Induction: Hand Clasp Induction (aka Modified Steeple Induction)

Clinician: Clasp your hands together but keep the index fingers straight and separated by 2 or 3 centimeters. Stare at the space between the fingers. As you stare, you will become aware of the fingers wanting to move together. Perhaps you have already noticed that the room is becoming more and more blurry as you focus between the fingers. As the fingers move together, you will become aware of your eyes feeling more strained. You can allow your eyes to close and your hands to drop comfortably to the lap when the tips of the index fingers finally meet. Just allow the fingers all the time they want. Sometimes they will move together quickly, sometimes it takes a few seconds.

[I originally learned this technique from Dr. Patrick McCarthy (Gow, 2011; see also Cyna, 2017). I find that it is a rapid technique and can work well in pain management situations in both adults and children. Suggestions should be given on the subject's outward breath and the subject instructed to close his or her eyes when the fingers meet, if this does not happen spontaneously. Due to the position of hands and tendons, the subject would have to actively resist the natural tendency for the fingers to move together. If the fingers do not move together, it may be that the subject has some reservations about being hypnotized.]

Special Place

Clinician: Imagine that you are walking towards a very inviting looking door. Behind this door is a special place that your imagination is already creating for you. It may be a place that you recognize having been to before, or it may be a place entirely new. Perhaps it is a mix of both. Allow this place to be exactly the place you want it to be.

It will be a safe place where you feel relaxed and at ease. You will feel freedom, peace, comfort, joy, relaxed, and rested. Notice the color of the door and whether the door has panels or is plain. Be aware of whether there is a door handle, and notice if it seems like the door will open towards or away from you. Take all the time you need, and when you are ready open the door and enter your special place.

As you take a few more steps into this place, notice how it becomes more and more vivid. It is as if it is in high definition. It is amazing. Notice what you can see and then what you can hear and smell and touch.

Take all the time you need to explore and enjoy this place. If you are outside, you may notice what time of day it is by the position of the sun and the time of year by the weather or any plants and trees you can see.

You will find that it is quite easy to talk. Tell me, what can you see in this place, where are you? Can you hear anything? Are there any smells or tastes? If you reach out, what can you touch? Excellent, now take a moment or two to find the perfect place in your special place to relax while you let your mind wonder.

[Ensure that you avoid inserting your own ideas into the patient's special place. If they explain that they have arrived at the beach, you should ask them to describe it, rather than assume it is a sandy beach in a hot place. Their special place beach may be a pebble beach in the rain! Be specifically vague, using statements such as, "It is the perfect beach, on the perfect day." Allow the patient to fill in the details. If the patient has already described their special place to you, or when they describe it during the session, use their words as you continue to talk about the place.]

Professor Dabney Ewin talks about changing the terminology of special place to laughing place (Ewin, 2009, p. 55). His concern is that special place may have underlying sexual connotations for some, which may provoke abreaction. Others use the term favorite place.

Dr. Patrick McCarthy has a version of the special place called The Special Place of Bliss (described in Frederick, 2001). This variation is well worth the effort to learn, as not only does it help patients enter hypnosis and relax, it also helps them deal with any unwanted emotions or thoughts in a non-intrusive way by offloading stones, which represent their worries and problems prior to passing through the doorway and entering the special place.

General dissociation could be considered as the ability to create a sense of complete dissociation from reality. This can be a very powerful pain control technique. Absorbing a patient fully in a special place so that they experience a strong sense of dissociation can have a profound effect on their ability to reduce pain. In a case where I am controlling pain using hypnosis as the main method of pain control, I will always therefore spend plenty of time in helping the patient become fully absorbed and to feel as dissociated as possible.

Dissociation can be enhanced by focusing in on minute details. Statements can be made about noticing the different color of each grain of sand, leaf, pebble, etc. The patient can be asked to "…enjoy the way the sunlight dances on the surface of the water." Be aware that the place need not necessarily be a relaxing place in order to produce dissociation.

So long as the patient can fully absorb themselves in the thought of being there it will be effective. They may choose to go skiing or jogging for example. These types of scenes can be useful when working with blood phobia or the vasovagal category of needle phobia (as the patient is stimulated and thus less likely to faint). In my experience, when it comes to pain control, most patients prefer to feel relaxed during dental procedures and so will choose relaxing places such as the beach, the woods, a walk in the mountains, their garden, a park, or their own bedroom, etc.

Deepening and Ego Strengthening

What follows is based on the "Calm, control, and confident" mantra using a triangle, adapted from a technique described by Craig et al. (1982). The script is for a visualizer and should be tailored as required. This technique is best incorporated into the patient's special place. In this example, we assume this is a beach. The triangle and words, however, may be drawn on any object, with any object.

Clinician: *Imagine* **that you are on your sandy beach and can see the sand below your feet.… When you can see this, just let me know by allowing your right index finger to move…** *[Prompt until finger moves. If it fails to move even following further prompting, continue with:]*

If you are unable to see this, can you imagine what it would be like if you could see it?

[To imagine that you can see the sand, and to imagine what it would be like if you could imagine that you can see the sand, are essentially the same concept. It always amazes me, however, when a patient is struggling to visualize something, that they will accept that they can imagine what it would be like if they could and are then happy to proceed. If, despite this, the patient is still having trouble, I would simply then state:]

That's OK. Just relax then and listen, because we are just going to consider some words.

Very good. **Now, imagine that with a stick or a shell or perhaps with just your finger you can draw a triangle in the sand.... That's right, very good. Hear the sounds as you draw the triangle** *[Engaging an auditory experience].* **Now, around the triangle, at its corners, you will write some words... starting at the top... with the word... CALM.** *See the letters as you spell out the word C... A... L... M...*

[See and C are both emphasized slightly in your intonation. The word CALM is spelled out slowly to aid deepening and is paced with each outward breath.]

Notice how the sand feels as you write the word CALM with the stick *[Engaging a kinesthetic experience].*

Just *allow* **yourself this feeling of CALM...**

[The word allow *is permissive and also creates a sense of deserving this reward. As children we are allowed treats like candy or staying up late at the weekend!]*

Enjoy **this feeling... from now on feeling** *calmer and calmer* **every day... every day feeling** *calmer and calmer...* **more and more** *calm...* **more** *optimistic...* **these feelings of calmness** *growing* and *increasing...* *calmer* and *calmer...* more *composed...* more at *peace... calm...* C... A... L... M...

Optional "Confusion Technique"

Clinician: Now, choose one of the remaining corners of the triangle... *or allow it to choose you...* the corner by which you would like to *write* the second word. If you choose the *right*, that's *alright*, if you chose the *left*, then the *right* is all that's *left, left* behind, but that's *alright* too. It's your *right* to *write* on the *left* or the *right*. To *write* on the *right* or the *left* is *right*. If it is the *left* corner, then that's all *right...* the *right* will be *left* for later... but *right* now <u>you will write</u>, and so as you do so <u>you will feel more and more relaxed</u> as you <u>now write the word CONTROL</u>.... C... O... N... T... R... O... L... [*Pace to outward breaths*] CONTROL.

And so, as you *write* the word *control*, it's *right* to <u>feel yourself more and more in control</u>.

> [*As the underlined parts make more sense after the confusion, it is easier for the subconscious to accept these suggestions.*]

As you become *calmer...* more *composed...* and more *confident...* more able to *cope...* you will find that you are *increasingly* able to... *control* your own life... each and every day from now on you will feel more and more in *control...* more in control of your *circumstances...* more in control of any *situation...* more in *control of yourself.* You will *enjoy* this new found *control...* this will allow you to *cope* with many situations... in exactly the way you want to.

The final word... to be written at the final corner... is the word... *CONFIDENT...* C... O... N... F... I... D... E... N... T... [*Pace to outward breaths*] **Confident.**

Confident to do the things that you *want* to do... *every day* feeling more and more *confident*... confident in *yourself*... confident in your *abilities*... confident in your *talents*... confident that you can become *CALM*...

Confident that you are in *control*, confident that you can become more *CONFIDENT!* In so doing, you can feel an increased ability to COPE. And as you write the word cope in the center of the triangle, you can feel an increased ability to cope grow within you. C... O... P... E... *[Pace to outward breaths]* Cope.

Read these words to yourself again. These words that you have written which all begin with "C"... and you will *now* begin to *see*... and *feel* and *hear* what these words *really* mean... CALM... CONTROL... CONFIDENT... COPE... *feel* how *powerful* these words are... CALM... CONTROL... CONFIDENT... COPE.

Glove Anesthesia/Glove Analgesia

The following script is one way of creating glove anesthesia and is a very useful technique in managing acute and chronic pain alike. As with any pain control technique, I usually give a suggestion that, "I would like to teach you a technique that many people have found to be very useful and effective. As with any hypnotic pain control technique that you will learn, it will only work if the pain has no *signal value* or purpose."

It is important that the hypnotist's technique is flexible and adapted to each individual case. The goal of glove anesthesia is that an alteration in sensation is achieved. The altered sensation will differ from person to person and indeed may vary in an individual at different appointments. It may be coldness, numbness, stiffness, tightness, etc. What is important is that the altered sensation is created and described by the patient.

The hypnotist should repeat the patient's own words when describing and amplifying the changes in sensation. I have found scripts for glove anesthesia that I have read in the past have been too focused on attempting to create a sensation of coldness, for example. While it may be effective to do this, some patients simply do not experience coldness during the technique or indeed they may dislike the feeling. Over the years, I have therefore adapted a more permissive script to allow the patient to experience glove anesthesia in whatever way is right for them.

[The hand should be positioned with the elbow supported, the forearm slightly raised, and the wrist limp with the hand drooping. This physical position will aid in the creation of an altered sensation.]

Clinician: Focus your attention on <u>your</u> right hand... and as you focus on <u>your</u> hand... pay attention to the tension in <u>the</u> hand... and notice how <u>the</u> hand feels and how <u>the</u> hand can begin to change.

[Notice that only the first two references to the hand are your. *The shift from* your *to* the *is important as it assists dissociation.]*

You will notice the feeling in the hand changing. It may happen quickly or it may take a few moments.

[You will is assertive. It can be said with some conviction, as the physical positioning of the hand will indeed create some change in the feeling. It may is permissive, however. This is followed by the bind happen quickly or it may take a few moments. *Success is assumed, whether it is quick or takes a few moments.]*

You may feel that the hand begins to feel colder. It may begin to feel more rubbery, or dull. Perhaps it will feel tingly—like pins and needles. I wonder what sensation you will experience.

[Again, this is an example of a bind, or what is sometimes known as an illusion of choice.]

Notice where in the hand you notice these altered feelings happening first. Is it the thumb? Or the pinky? The front of the hand, or the back?

[The word first *assumes that it will happen elsewhere next. The list of options is again an illusion of choice.]*

Can you feel it changing yet?

[The word yet *here implies that if the answer is currently no, then the patient will feel it change at some point.]*

What does it feel like?

[This question is important as it allows the clinician to begin to repeat back the exact descriptive words used by the patient to then strengthen the experience.]

Yes... that's right, it feels... *[repeat the patient's description].*

[This gives reassurance that they are doing the right thing and the praise you give strengthens the experience and the speed of progress.]

Notice how that is feeling really... *[repeat patient's description]* and how that allows the hand to feel comfortable and insensitive.

Where is that feeling the strongest and most powerful?

Allow it to spread now.

I wonder if it will stop at the wrist or travel a little further up the arm. Feel how *[repeat patient's description]* the hand becomes now, how insensitive.

That's good. Now, in a moment the hand will become so... *[repeat patient's description]* and insensitive... that when I pinch the back of the hand... you can be pleasantly surprised by just how insensitive it really is. And as that process continues in its own time... and in its own way... the hand can continue to become more and more insensitive... and you can enjoy noticing that insensitivity in the hand... and how different it can be from <u>your</u> other hand.

[Note the reversion to your other hand, as this other hand does not have altered sensation or a sense of dissociation.

Glove anesthesia can be easily transferred between hands. The patient is asked to touch their hands together and suggestions are given that they can take all the time they need in the next few minutes to allow the altered sensation(s) to transfer to the other hand. Once this has been demonstrated successfully, the patient can then be instructed to transfer the altered sensation(s) to any other part of their body (such as a tooth) to alleviate or manage pain. Remember, it is essential that any altered sensation(s) be returned to normal by the end of the session, unless long-term pain management at a specific site is required.

Patients vary in ability with this technique. For some, the first attempt may produce only a slight difference in sensation, while for others, the effect will be a complete loss of feeling. It is, however, important to reverse it, even if the effect is slight.]

Now, you are doing really well... and in the future... I'm sure you will be really pleased to discover... every time you wish to allow the hand [or the body part transferred to] to become insensitive and [insert patient's description] like this... it can happen more strongly... powerfully and rapidly.

So, now it is time to allow the sensations in <u>your</u> hand [or other body part] to return to normal... with full comfort.... As you move or shake your hands and fingers now you can notice how all normal sensations return to your hand. Notice how it can happen quickly or can take a few moments. Back to normal. Well done.

Glove anesthesia can be produced or amplified by a variety of suggestions.

1. Altered sensation in the chosen hand can be increased by referring to it as *the* hand, rather than *your* hand.

2. Direct suggestions such as, "As I stroke the hand you will notice the hand becoming more and more numb/cold/etc.," or "As I lift each finger in turn you can notice the fingers becoming number and stiffer" can be useful.

3. Imagery suited to the patient's description of the altered sensation, such as immersion of the hand into ice cold water, holding a cold glass of their favorite drink, putting on a heavy protective or rubber glove, rubbing in a magic numbing cream, etc. can also be very effective.

4. The *magic spot* technique involves the transfer of feeling into another object, for example a large coin from the area it contacts.

5. Draining away suggestion: "As I lift your arm up now, *[lift hand and arm vertically up]* imagine that any remaining normal feelings in the hand are draining away, down the arm, leaving it colder and number... insensitive... comfortable... and twice as numb... and twice as insensitive as before... colder and number... you can really enjoy noticing that insensitivity in the hand... and how it can feel very different from your other hand."

6. This technique requires the patient to imagine that the body area in question (e.g., the hand) has detached from their body or "floated away somewhere else." The suggestion can be given that the hand can be "a part of you, but apart from you... like a mannequin hand."

7. Suggestions can also be given for complete separation from pain. The patient can imagine going somewhere else, leaving his/her body behind while engaging in something more enjoyable or interesting. Immersion or focus on a special place can effectively create this general feeling of dissociation from the entire body even during a technique such as glove anesthesia.

8. Memory can be used to create hypnoanesthesia to control pain. For example, "Do you recall the last time you felt the numbness of a local anesthetic? Do you remember that feeling of numbness, thickness, fullness? Describe to me what it would feel like if you now had that numb feeling in your mouth/body. As you think about those feelings, allow the memory of them to allow that feeling to grow comfortably stronger. Do you also recall how comfortable it is to

have a procedure once the area is numb? As you create this feeling of numbness, you can be confident that the procedure to improve your health can be carried out in total comfort.

9. Always give the patient objective proof of the anesthesia; for example, by pinching the skin on the back of the hand.

10. Once the procedure has been completed, a post hypnotic suggestion can be given that: "This altered feeling will last the same length of time that it would normally last if you had had a local anesthetic. As the sensation gradually wears off over the next few hours, you will be surprised by how comfortable the area feels and how quickly everything heals."

The Comfort Dial

This technique has the advantage that you are able to also monitor the patient's subjective assessment of pain on an ongoing basis, simply by asking them what number the dial is currently at throughout a procedure.

Clinician: Many people can alter their experience of comfort by using something called the comfort dial. So, in a few moments you will begin to create your own personal comfort dial. It will be a gauge that will indicate your level of comfort or discomfort, from 0 to 10.

Notice how the numbers 0 to 10 are marked on the dial. Zero is totally comfortable and 10 is discomfort or pain. This gauge will also have the ability to be controlled by you. Some people imagine a dial that is like a thermostat. Others imagine the volume control on a stereo, or the controls of a shower. It may be the speedometer on a car, or it can be like

the dial on a safe. Whatever feels correct is right for you. Create your comfort dial now and describe to me what it is like.

Acute Pain Case

Clinician: As the work gets underway that will make your mouth healthier, you can remind yourself that everything that can be done to help you become healthier is now happening, and for that reason, it is reasonable to turn the dial down. Zero in on the dial as you turn the dial down.

[During the procedure, the concept of turning the dial down is repeated.]

Chronic Pain Case

Clinician: Notice what number the dial is at right now. With your permission, I'd like to demonstrate the control you have over the dial by asking you to turn the dial up, just for a moment. Notice how by focusing on the discomfort, you can amplify it. And then turn the dial back down again so that it is only a [insert original number].

[After repeating two or three times,] and so as you can turn the dial up, you can now turn the dial down. Do that now. Turn the dial down to a number that you feel will allow you to get on with your life. Tell me when you have achieved that.

Basic Imagery Techniques

1. Pain can be identified as an electric current, and the patient can be asked to imagine that they have a set of switches. The circuit can be switched off at certain points to prevent the current from travelling up and down.

2. Similarly, a patient may identify with the gate control theory in terms of a telephone switchboard, with pain defined as messages passing up and down. They can choose to unplug cables or switch off the telephone.

Reversal Script

Clinician: In the future, you will find it easier to go into trance at appropriate and safe times for you to do so and with your full knowledge and prior consent. Hypnosis for pain control will be effective only when there is a reason or justification for it. Hypnosis should only be considered for pain control following all appropriate assessments and investigations. You will only allow yourself to be hypnotized during your self-hypnosis sessions or with the guidance of a medical doctor, dentist, psychologist, or other appropriate professional who is trained in the use of hypnosis.

Reversal/Arousal/Re-orientation

Traditional reverse-counting techniques are often disliked by patients as it assumes that they will respond and re-orientate exactly in time with the counting, which is a problem encountered surprisingly frequently. A more permissive and gentle way would be the following.

Clinician: And now it is time to fully return to the present moment; back fully present in your physical body. Any altered sensations that are useful, you can keep for now. However, they will gradually soften and disappear. So, any strange sensations… totally disappearing.

Your muscle tone returns to normal. Your coordination returns to normal. And this will happen each time you come out of trance.

Bright, alert, and wide awake.

When you are ready... open your eyes.

Well done.

Self-Hypnosis

Whichever technique is preferred by the patient, it is important that they learn how to utilize it themselves with their self-hypnosis. This allows patients the ability to create the effect themselves prior to their appointment. The patient should be taught how to use the comfort dial, achieve glove anesthesia, and transfer it using self-hypnosis. This ability for the patient to have ownership of and easy access to the techniques is empowering and is an important factor in their long-term success.

References

Chaves. J. F. (1997). Hypnosis in dentistry: Historical overview and current appraisal. In M. Mehrstedt & P. O. Wikstrom (Eds.), *Hypnosis in dentistry: Hypnosis International Monographs 3* (pp. 5-23). Munich, Germany: MEG Stiftung.

Craig, S., Fairful-Smith, G. W., & Ferguson, M. M. (1982, August). *The treatment of Apthous Stomatitis and Lichen Planus with hypnotherapy.* Paper presented at the Ninth International Congress of Hypnosis and Psychosomatic Medicine, Glasgow, Scotland.

Cyna, A. M. (2017). The modified steeple technique and the GR Wicks induction. In M. P. Jensen, *The art and practice of hypnotic induction: Favorite methods of master clinicians* (pp. 256-267). Kirkland, WA: Denny Creek Press.

Ewin, D. M. (2009). *101 things I wish I'd known when I started using hypnosis*. Bancyfelin, United Kingdom: Crown House Publishing.

Frederick, L. E. (2001). The use of hypnosis in surgery and anaesthesiology: Psychological preparation of the surgical patient. Springfield, IL: Charles C. Thomas.

Gow, M. A. (2006a). Hypnosis with a 31-year-old female with dental phobia requiring emergency extraction. *Contemporary Hypnosis, 23*, 83-91.

Gow, M. A. (2006b). Hypnosis with a blind 55-year-old female with dental phobia requiring periodontal treatment and extraction. *Contemporary Hypnosis, 23*, 92-100.

Gow, M. A. (2008). Are you positive? *Dentistry, 9*, 23–25.

Gow, M. A. (2010). Dental extractions and immediate implant placements using hypnosis in place of traditional local anesthetics. *Contemporary Hypnosis, 27*, 268–277.

Gow, M. A. (2011). Hypnosis in dentistry. In A. Weiner (Ed.), *The fearful dental patient: A guide to understanding and managing* (pp. 139-171). Ames, IA: Wiley-Blackwell.

Gow, M. A., & Faqir, A. (2008). Internal sinus lift and placement of an osseointegrated implant using hypnosis as the sole method of pain control – a first in dental practice. *Implant Dentistry Today, 2*, 31-37

Kane, S., & Olness, K. (2004). *The art of therapeutic communication: The collected works of Kay Thompson*. Williston, VT: Crown House.

Stolzenburg, J. (1961). Technique in conditioning and hypnosis for control of gagging. *International Journal of Clinical and Experimental Hypnosis, 9*, 97-104.

Thompson, K. F. (1963). A rationale for suggestion in dentistry. *American Journal of Clinical Hypnosis, 5*, 181-186.

Thompson, K. F. (1977). Hypnosis in dental practice. In M. Weisenberg (Ed.), *The control of pain.* New York, NY: Psychological Dimensions.

For Further Reading...

Brann, L., Owens, J., & Williamson, A. (2012). *The handbook of contemporary clinical hypnosis.* Chichester, United Kingdom: Wiley-Blackwell.

Brown, D. C. (2009). *Advances in the use of hypnosis for medicine, dentistry and pain prevention/management.* Carmathen, United Kingdom: Crown House Publishing.

Simons, D., Potter C., & Temple, G. (2007). *Hypnosis and communication in dental practice.* Surry, United Kingdom: Quintessence Publishing.

Yapko, M. D. (2003) *Trancework* (4th ed.). New York, NY: Brunner-Routledge.

ABOUT THE EDITOR

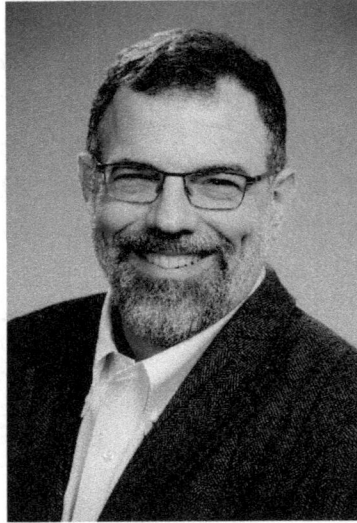

Mark P. Jensen, PhD, is a Professor and Vice Chair for Research at the Department of Rehabilitation Medicine, University of Washington, in Seattle, Washington, USA. He has been studying chronic pain and helping individuals effectively manage pain for over 30 years. He has been funded by the National Institutes of Health and other funding agencies to study the efficacy and mechanisms of different treatments for chronic pain, including hypnosis. He has published extensively (seven books and over 500 articles and book chapters) on the topics of pain assessment and treatment.

He has received numerous awards for his writing and scientific contributions including: the Jay Haley Early Career

Award for Innovative Contributions to Hypnosis from the International Society of Hypnosis, the Clark L. Hull Award for Scientific Excellence in Writing on Experimental Hypnosis from the *American Journal of Clinical Hypnosis*, the Wilbert E. Fordyce Clinical Investigator Award from the American Pain Society, and both the Distinguished Contributions to Scientific Hypnosis and Distinguished Contributions Professional Hypnosis Awards from the American Psychological Association Division 30, among others.

His book on the use of hypnosis for chronic pain management (*Hypnosis for Chronic Pain Management: Therapist Guide*, published by Oxford University Press) won the 2011 Society for Clinical and Experimental Hypnosis Arthur Shapiro Award: Best Book on Hypnosis. He is also a popular international speaker and workshop facilitator.

CPSIA information can be obtained
at www.ICGtesting.com
Printed in the USA
BVHW071734100521
606946BV00004B/581